18.90

infertility:
the hidden causes

how to overcome them naturally

Sandra Cabot MD
Margaret Jasinska ND

D0910833

Infertility: the hidden causes

Copyright © 2011 Sandra Cabot MD & Margaret Jasinska ND

Published by WHAS Pty Ltd
PO Box 689 Camden NSW Australia 2570
Phone 02 4655 8855

Edited and reprinted for the United States of America in 2011
Published by SCB International Inc. - United States of America
PO Box 5070 Glendale AZ USA 85312 Phone 623 334 3232

www.liverdoctor.com
www.weightcontroldoctor.com.au
www.sandracabot.com

USA Paperback ISBN: 978-0-9673983-4-1

1) Infertility 2) Nutrition 3) Natural Therapies 4) Pregnancy

Contents

Introduction

One in six couples struggles with infertility. Among women over the age of 35, one in three experience difficulties conceiving. Fertility problems are escalating and it's not just women in their late 30s that are affected. Infertility is a sign that something is not right with you or your partner's health. A healthy body is a fertile body. Our bodies are cleverly designed to reproduce, and when that doesn't happen, there is always an explanation.

No organ system in your body operates in isolation. The health of your reproductive system is enormously influenced by your immune system, your digestive system, your liver, your thyroid gland and your emotional state, just to name a few. Mother Nature is wise, and if there are areas of your body that are not in optimum health, it is not in your interest to become pregnant. Pregnancy is an enormous stress on a woman's body and your body needs to be in optimal health or very close to it in order to achieve a healthy pregnancy and healthy baby. Of course, you may know several unhealthy couples, with terrible diets who have had problem free pregnancies and healthy children. These people will always exist, just like heavy drinkers and chain smokers who die peacefully in their sleep in their 90s! These people are the lucky few who are the exception to the rule. Our aim in writing this book is not just to get you pregnant, although this book will greatly increase your chances, but it is also designed to optimize your chances of a healthy, problem free pregnancy and healthy children.

Being diagnosed with infertility is extremely distressing and it may leave you feeling confused and hopeless. We have written this book to educate you about the dozens of seemingly unrelated and often overlooked factors that may be compromising your fertility. Knowledge is power, and the more you understand about your body, the better able you will be to make decisions.

The use of IVF and other assisted reproductive technologies has skyrocketed in recent decades. Currently one percent of all children born in the USA are conceived through the use of these technologies. While it's wonderful that IVF is available and can help many couples achieve their dream of having a family, we believe the technology is very over used and not without risks. IVF was originally designed to overcome plumbing problems; basically where tubal problems prevented the egg and sperm from being able to join. However, these days it is used for any and every case of infertility, often without properly investigating the underlying cause of the problem. This is sad because these causes are often easily overcome as you will learn in this book.

Typically your doctor will organise a handful of blood tests, perhaps a pelvic ultrasound and sometimes other tests. If everything comes back normal, you will probably be labeled with unexplained infertility. But does that really mean your infertility is unexplained, or just that your doctor has failed to find an explanation? And is that a justified reason to begin the expensive and emotional journey of IVF? What if your thyroid gland is responsible for your inability to conceive or causing you to miscarry? What if a vitamin D deficiency is preventing you from ovulating? Or perhaps your allergies are clogging your fallopian tubes with mucus, thus preventing your partner's sperm from joining your egg? Don't you think it's essential to rule out every known possible and treatable cause of infertility before resorting to IVF?

Male infertility is rising just as quickly as female infertility. Your partner may have a low sperm count and high levels of abnormal sperm. You probably haven't been offered a lot of solutions to correct this; you may even have been told it's genetic and nothing can be done, so IVF is your only option. Sperm counts in the average healthy man have more than halved in the last 50 years; so much so that one in 25 men is now considered infertile. The average man today is lucky if 15 percent of the sperm he produces have a normal shape. Such rapid and dramatic drops in sperm quality and quantity cannot be explained by genes. Sperm are more susceptible to harm caused by environmental chemicals and nutrient deficiencies than eggs, and we will explain the most effective ways to boost male fertility.

In this book we cover the common and obvious causes of infertility, such as polycystic ovarian syndrome and endometriosis, as well as the subtle, often overlooked causes of infertility. It's a sad fact that scientists know more about how diet affects fertility in livestock animals than the average doctor knows about diet and fertility in humans. We have spent several years researching the topics in this book and sincerely hope the information contained within will help solve the infertility puzzle for you. The healthier both you and your partner are, the better quality your egg and sperm will be. The genetic material inside the egg and sperm form the basis of your child's lifelong health. By optimizing the health of you, the parents, we hope to create a healthier future generation.

1. How common is infertility and what causes it?

Infertility is an increasingly common problem in the USA; it affects one in six couples. The definition of infertility is an inability for a couple to conceive after 12 months of unprotected intercourse, or the inability to carry a pregnancy to a live birth. [1.] If a woman is 35 years of age or older, the couple is considered infertile if they have been trying to conceive for six months or longer. Infertility is an escalating problem worldwide; the World Health Organization estimates that 80 million people in the world are infertile. Infertility is not always caused by a problem with a woman; male infertility is becoming increasingly common. It is estimated that 40 percent of infertility cases are due to factors in the woman; 40 to 50 percent are due to male factors, and 15 to 20 percent of cases are due to factors in both partners. Women over the age of 35 are twice as likely to suffer with infertility as younger women.

A number of factors can be responsible for infertility. A couple may be affected by one of these factors, or by a combination of them. The most common causes of male and female infertility are listed in the table below. Each of the causes will be explained fully later in this book, along with our recommendations for overcoming them. When treating infertility we need to look beyond the reproductive tract; we need to look at the entire body. In many cases health problems that you think have nothing to do with your reproductive tract are in fact responsible for your infertility.

Female causes of infertility

- Ovulation disorders
- Polycystic ovarian syndrome
- Tubal problems
- Endometriosis
- Premature menopause
- Infections

- Hormonal problems
- Repeated miscarriage
- Immune system and blood clotting disorders
- Uterine fibroids and polyps
- Exposure to chemicals
- Poor nutrition
- Age
- Stress

Male causes of infertility

- Low sperm count or abnormal sperm
- Tubal problems
- Exposure to excessive heat
- Exposure to chemicals
- Hormonal problems
- Testicular problems
- Functional problems, including erectile dysfunction and retrograde ejaculation
- Immune system disorders
- Infections
- Poor nutrition
- Age

In up to 20 percent of couples medical tests cannot determine a concrete cause for infertility and it is deemed "unexplained".

2. The female reproductive system explained

Before we explain the causes and treatment of infertility in great detail, we will explain the basics of the reproductive system and conception so that you are familiar with various terms.

Conception occurs when an egg from a woman is fertilized by a sperm from a man. Eggs are referred to as ova and they are made in the ovaries. Sperm are produced in the testicles. Ovaries and testicles are also referred to as gonads and they produce sex hormones.

The female reproductive system

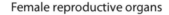

Female reproductive organs

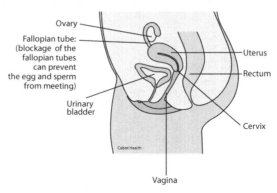

Ovary
Fallopian tube: (blockage of the fallopian tubes can prevent the egg and sperm from meeting)
Urinary bladder
Uterus
Rectum
Cervix
Cabot Health
Vagina

The two ovaries are roughly the size of almonds and they produce ova (eggs) as well as the hormones estrogen and progesterone. We say the ovaries produce eggs, but to be more specific, the eggs mature and ripen inside the ovaries. The ovaries contain ovarian follicles, which is where eggs develop. The eggs develop inside the ovaries while a woman is a fetus inside her mother's uterus. When a baby girl is born, she already has approximately two million eggs. This means the quality of the eggs inside your ovaries is dependent on your mother's diet and lifestyle while she was pregnant with you. Throughout life, many ovarian follicles break down and get reabsorbed by the body, so by the time a girl reaches puberty and her menstrual cycle begins; only approximately 400, 000 ovarian follicles are left to develop into mature eggs.

The ovaries are held in place by ligaments that connect them to the uterus and pelvis. The uterus (womb) is a pear shaped organ that is the size of a fist, but stretches when a woman is pregnant. The thick wall of the uterus is made of three layers. The inner lining of the uterus is called the endometrium. The endometrium is shed during menstruation. When a woman becomes pregnant, the endometrium thickens and is filled with blood vessels that eventually develop into the placenta. The deeper layer of the uterus contains powerful muscles that contract during labor to push the baby down the birth canal (vagina). The outermost layer of the uterus consists of tissue that helps to hold it in place in the pelvis. The lower third of the uterus is called the cervix. The cervix extends down to the vagina.

The fallopian tubes (also called oviducts) are approximately 10 centimeters long and they connect the ovaries to the uterus. The fallopian tubes have finger-like projections on their ends at the ovaries. When an egg is released by an ovary, the finger-like projections catch it and transport it down the fallopian tube and to the uterus. It takes an egg approximately five days to travel from the ovary to the uterus. Fertilization occurs when an egg meets a sperm during its journey down the fallopian tube. An egg only lives for approximately 24 hours after it leaves an ovary, therefore fertilization usually occurs in the upper third portion of a fallopian tube.

The female menstrual cycle

The menstrual cycle is divided into two phases: the follicular phase and the luteal phase. The follicular phase begins on the first day of menstruation and ends at ovulation. The luteal phase begins at ovulation and ends when menstrual bleeding begins.

The follicular phase

The levels of estrogen and progesterone in a woman's body are at their lowest just before a menstrual period begins. This causes two things to happen; firstly the lining of the uterus starts to shed. This causes menstrual bleeding. If you are counting the days of your cycle, day one is the first day bleeding begins. The other thing that happens is the pituitary gland in the brain begins to increase its production of the hormone called FSH (Follicle Stimulating Hormone). FSH stimulates ovarian follicles (eggs in their sacs) to begin maturing in the ovaries.

FSH causes between 10 and 20 ovarian follicles to start maturing, but only one (occasionally two) will mature fully. As the ovarian follicles grow and mature, they produce increasing amounts of estrogen, which stimulates the uterine lining to grow and thicken, in preparation for fertilization. Estrogen also causes the cervical mucus to develop a thinner consistency, aiding the passage of sperm through the cervix. The follicular phase of menstruation typically lasts between 10 and 14 days, but it can vary enormously in length. It gets shorter as a woman approaches menopause.

Ovulation

When the estrogen produced by the ovarian follicles reaches a high enough level, it triggers the pituitary gland in the brain to release a surge of LH (Luteinizing Hormone). This causes the most mature follicle inside the ovary to burst open and release its egg into the fallopian tube. That is ovulation and it usually occurs 14 days before the next menstrual period. The few days before ovulation are considered a woman's most fertile time. This is because sperm typically survive for three to four days inside a woman's body (but can sometimes survive for up to seven days). If a woman has sexual intercourse up to seven days before she ovulates, it is possible for the sperm to still be alive inside her when she ovulates, leading to fertilization. A woman is still considered fertile one or two days after ovulation because the egg typically lives for 24 hours after ovulation. From a few days after she has ovulated, up to her next menstrual bleed, a woman is considered not fertile.

The luteal phase

The time from ovulation until the next menstrual period is the luteal phase. This phase usually lasts between 12 and 16 days. The luteal phase tends to be more constant than the follicular phase; so whether you have a long, normal or short cycle, the luteal phase generally remains between 12 and 16 days long. After the egg has been released at ovulation, the empty follicle changes structure and becomes known as the corpus luteum (meaning white body). The corpus luteum produces progesterone, and it continues to produce smaller amounts of estrogen.

Progesterone causes the lining of the uterus to produce nourishing fluids, just in case the egg becomes fertilized and implants itself in the endometrium (lining of the uterus). If fertilization does occur, the corpus luteum continues to produce progesterone for approximately the first eight weeks of pregnancy; after that time the placenta develops and it takes over the task of progesterone production. Adequate progesterone production is vitally important in the early stages of pregnancy, and lack of progesterone is a common cause of early miscarriage, (as well as inability to conceive in the first place).

If fertilization does not occur, the empty follicle (corpus luteum) starts to break down and eventually stops producing hormones. When the corpus luteum stops all hormone production, the lining of the uterus is shed and that heralds the beginning of another menstrual bleed.

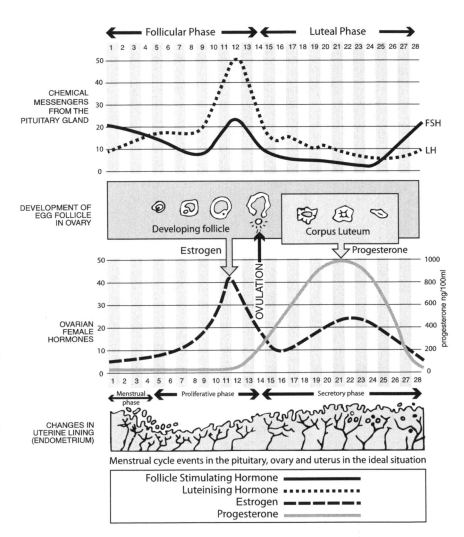

Menstrual cycle events in the pituitary, ovary and uterus in the ideal situation

Follicle Stimulating Hormone	━━━━━━━
Luteinising Hormone	••••••••••
Estrogen	━ ━ ━ ━ ━
Progesterone	▨▨▨▨▨▨

Determining your most fertile time

The ideal time for conception

Counting the days of your menstrual cycle can help you determine how regular your cycles are and the day you are likely to ovulate. This will help you determine when you are most fertile, and therefore when sexual intercourse is most likely to result in conception. A normal menstrual cycle is between 23 and 35 days. Cycles that are shorter or longer than this can be caused by a variety of factors, but they indicate that ovulation is probably not occurring. If there is no ovulation, there can obviously not be any fertilization. According to Chanley Small, Ph.D, researcher and reproductive epidemiologist at Emory University in the USA, women with 30 to 31 day cycles are the most fertile. Women with cycles shorter than 28 days are more likely to produce eggs of poorer quality.

To determine how long your cycle is, use the following method. Day one of your cycle is the day menstrual bleeding begins. Continue counting until the day before your next menstrual period begins. If your period began on 1st March and your next period started on 29th March, you have a 28 day cycle. Plot your menstrual period on a calendar for at least 3 months to get an average length for your cycle. Your cycle can vary in length slightly from month to month and that is usually not a problem.

In a 28 day cycle ovulation usually occurs on day 14. Women usually ovulate approximately 14 days before the start of menstrual bleeding.

Your most fertile time is during the two days before ovulation and one day afterwards.

All women are different and it is very imprecise to rely on the 14 day rule to indicate when you have ovulated. Luckily your body gives you several signs to indicate that ovulation has occurred. Getting familiar with these signs, and tracking them for several months can help you become in tune with your menstrual cycle, and optimize your chance of conception. Changes in your cervical mucus and basal body temperature are useful indicators of ovulation.

Cervical mucus

The quantity and type of mucus your cervix makes varies during your menstrual cycle. Paying attention to your mucus is an easy and fairly reliable way to determine where you are in your cycle. At the beginning of your menstrual cycle, estrogen levels are low, therefore very little mucus is produced. As you get closer to ovulation, mucus production increases; mucus may be sticky, white, cloudy or milky. This indicates you are approaching your fertile phase.

Just before ovulation, mucus becomes slippery, stretchy and clear; this is commonly referred to as raw egg white mucus, because that is what it resembles. The presence of this type of mucus signals the most fertile time in a woman's cycle. The egg white-type mucus facilitates the travel of sperm from the vagina, through the cervix, into the uterus and then fallopian tubes in search of an egg. Ovulation occurs one or two days after the development of this type of mucus. If you are trying to conceive it is recommended you have intercourse every day, beginning as soon as you detect egg white-type mucus.

After ovulation, mucus becomes thicker and cloudier. You may still be fertile during this stage, but only for two or three days at most. For the remainder of your cycle, the cervix produces mucus that is thick, sticky and acidic. The mucus stays around the opening of the cervix, acting to block the entry of sperm. Most women do not produce noticeable quantities of mucus at this stage, and feel more dry than at other times of their cycle.

You can check the type of mucus your cervix makes by looking for a discharge left on your underpants or toilet paper, or by inserting a clean finger into your vagina. Egg white type fertile mucus will stretch several centimeters between your fingers and it will look clear and mucus-like. Normally, you should only notice this type of fertile mucus once in your cycle, in the couple of days just before ovulation. A minority of women experience multiple batches of egg-white mucus during their menstrual cycle. This is common in women with polycystic ovarian syndrome. This condition is discussed in detail in chapter 3. Some women never notice appreciable changes in their cervical mucus throughout their cycle. In most cases this is not a problem and it is still possible to get pregnant despite this.

If your cervical mucus is constant, does not go through changes, is irritating, itchy or has an offensive smell, you probably have an infection and it is important to see your doctor.

What happens if there is no detectable cervical mucus?

Some women produce very little mucus and this reduces the chances of conception. The most common factors to affect cervical mucus production include:

- Anti-histamine use and the use of other anti-allergy medication.
- Some antibiotics.
- Clomiphene; a medication used to induce ovulation in infertile women.
- Cough suppressants
- Some cold and flu and sinus medication
- Other medication including sleeping tablets, atropine, propantheline, some anti-depressants and some epilepsy medication
- Age. Women in their 20s produce greater quantities of cervical mucus for more days than women over 35.
- Being underweight. This affects estrogen production; therefore less mucus is usually produced.
- Vaginal douching. Obviously this practice can wash away cervical mucus. Do not practice vaginal douching while attempting to conceive unless you are trying to overcome an infection and are under the guidance of a health care practitioner.
- Infection of the reproductive tract.
- Previous treatment for cervical cancer or pre-cancerous changes, such as cervical cone biopsy.
- Hormonal problems that result in anovulation (lack of ovulation). This is discussed in detail later in this chapter.
- Stress
- Previous D and C (dilation and curettage)

Sometimes adequate cervical mucus is produced, but the mucus is inhospitable to sperm. This is commonly referred to as having hostile mucus. The mucus does not allow the sperm to survive inside the female reproductive tract and impedes sperm transport. Mucus may be hostile for the following reasons:

- Poor quality mucus due to poor diet and nutritional deficiencies.
- Too acidic. Mucus can be too acidic due to the following factors: too much alcohol, sugar, dairy products, white flour, gluten and red meat. All of those foods have an acidic effect in the body, whereas fresh vegetables and fruit have an alkaline effect.
- Genitourinary infections produce hostile mucus.

- Food allergies can cause the production of excessively thick mucus that impedes the travel of sperm through the female reproductive tract.

Basal body temperature

Body at rest temperature

Another way of determining when you ovulate is by measuring your temperature when your body is at rest. This method is cumbersome and not entirely accurate, but it can be used as a backup, in combination with other methods. This method is more useful for women who have regular menstrual cycles that are close to 28 days long. You will need to measure your body temperature with a mercury thermometer first thing in the morning when you wake up, before getting out of bed. Your body temperature remains fairly constant each day under normal circumstances, however just after ovulation your temperature rises by 32.4 to 32.9 degrees Fahrenheit (0.2 to 0.5 degrees Celsius), and remains elevated until your next period. The rise in body temperature is caused by the progesterone released from the follicle after ovulation.

The basal body temperature test can tell you when you have already ovulated. It is often already too late to conceive once you've noticed that your temperature has risen; however if you take your temperature each day for several months you can watch for a pattern, and then plan intercourse in the day or two before your temperature is due to rise in subsequent menstrual cycles.

Women are most fertile the few days before their basal temperature rises, and are least fertile when their temperature has remained elevated more than three days.

Instructions for measuring your basal body temperature

Use a mercury thermometer, as they are more reliable than digital thermometers for measuring small changes in temperature. Take your temperature the same time each morning, as soon as you wake up, by placing the thermometer in your mouth. You should only take your temperature if you have had at least 4 hours of solid sleep before waking. So if you have had a restless night, or gone for a bathroom trip four hours before waking, this method will not be as reliable. That may exclude a lot of women! For accuracy, your temperature should be taken at the same time each morning. Sleeping in late on the weekend can make it more difficult to see a pattern and link temperature changes to ovulation.

Several things can affect your temperature, thus making this method inaccurate; these include an infection or other illness, stress, alcohol consumption the previous day, allergies, iron deficiency, adrenal gland exhaustion, thyroid disorders and some medication. If used on its own, the basal body temperature method of tracking ovulation is not always reliable.

If you notice a rise in your basal body temperature after ovulation, and your temperature has remained elevated for more than 20 days, this could indicate you are pregnant.

Ovulation monitoring kits

There are several fertility monitoring kits available on the market that are very helpful for determining the fertile days of your menstrual cycle. Most kits work by measuring luteinizing hormone (LH) levels in your urine. Immediately before ovulation, the body produces a large amount of luteinizing hormone, which triggers the release of a ripe egg from the ovary. Ovulation test kits detect a surge of luteinizing hormone in the urine, which indicates that ovulation will likely occur in the next 24 to 48 hours. This is your most fertile time and the optimum time for sexual intercourse that can lead to pregnancy. Ovulation monitoring kits are much less reliable in women with short or long cycles, or women with polycystic ovarian syndrome.

Some fertility monitoring kits measure estrogen levels in the saliva. These kits detect an increase in estrogen levels, approximately two to three days before ovulation. There is not as much evidence to support the accuracy of these kits.

Anovulation - failure to ovulate

A large percentage of women are not able to conceive because they do not ovulate, or don't ovulate regularly; this is called anovulation. Most women who do not ovulate have irregular menstrual cycles, and sometimes they don't menstruate at all for several months or years. If your menstrual cycles are shorter than 23 days, or longer than 35 days, you are probably not ovulating. If the length of your menstrual cycle varies greatly from month to month, that also indicates you are probably not ovulating. If you do not ovulate, your chances of getting pregnant in that month are zero because there is no egg to fertilize.

The most common causes of anovulation include:

- *Polycystic ovarian syndrome. This is by far the most common cause and will be discussed in detail in chapter 3*
- *Obesity*
- *Syndrome X (insulin resistance). You do not have to be overweight to have insulin resistance.*
- *Too low body weight*
- *Recent change in weight*
- *Illness*
- *Extreme exercise*
- *Hyperprolactinemia - i.e. High blood levels of the hormone prolactin. This is discussed in chapter 3*
- *Advancing maternal age; failure to ovulate is more common in women over 35*
- *Menopause and premature ovarian failure*
- *Disorders of the hypothalamus or pituitary gland in the brain*
- *Over or under active thyroid gland*
- *Stress. This is a big and underappreciated cause of anovulation.*
- *Iron deficiency*
- *Vitamin D deficiency*

The treatment of anovulation depends on the cause. Sometimes women who don't ovulate continue to experience a monthly bleed and sometimes they don't. This book addresses each of the causes of lack of ovulation and tells you what to do to overcome it. The most common medical treatment for anovulation is the fertility drug clomiphene (brand names Clomid and Serophene). There is more information about clomiphene and other prescription fertility medication in chapter 12

3. Hormonal Disorders that cause Infertility in women

Endometriosis

Endometriosis is one of the leading causes of infertility in women. The condition affects between 15 and 20 percent of women in their reproductive life,[2] while endometriosis is present in between 30 and 50 percent of women with infertility [3]. Endometriosis is a condition where the lining of the uterus (endometrium) grows outside of the uterus. Endometrial cells travel to the abdominal cavity and may attach themselves to the ovaries, fallopian tubes, behind the uterus, the bowel, bladder and other nearby structures. Rarely endometrial tissue travels to distant parts of the body. Each month the endometrial tissue builds up and then bleeds; although the blood is not able to leave the body with the menstrual flow if it is found in areas other than the uterus. Because the blood cannot escape, surrounding organs and tissues can stick to each other and form scar tissue.

Why is endometriosis so common?

There are several theories for the cause of endometriosis, but most authorities believe that it is an inflammatory disease, as it shares several features in common with autoimmune disease. Research has shown that anti-endometrial antibodies are present in 60 percent of endometriosis patients. All women with endometriosis have high levels of inflammatory chemicals in their bloodstream and they suffer with impaired immune system function. Endometriosis tends to run in families and environmental chemicals are also thought to play a big role in the disease. Researchers have been able to induce endometriosis in laboratory animals by exposing them to minute quantities of PCBs (polychlorinated biphenyls) and dioxins.[4] In one study scientists were able to cause endometriosis in monkeys with dioxin contaminated food, at precisely the dose that humans are commonly exposed to in the food supply.[5]

Research in humans has shown that blood levels of PCBs and DDE (the major breakdown product of DDT) are significantly higher in women with endometriosis than healthy women. It is thought that these chemicals cause detrimental changes in immune system function.[6] Environmental chemicals that compromise fertility are explained in detail in chapter 9.

Women who start menstruating young (younger than 12 years), and who experience very painful menstrual cramps early in life, tend to have the worst cases of endometriosis. It is also more common in women who bleed for longer than seven days, and women who have a menstrual cycle shorter than 27 days.

Signs and symptoms of endometriosis

The following list describes the main symptoms of endometriosis. Most women will not experience every symptom:

- Painful menstrual periods - immediately before and during bleeding
- Pain during and/or after sexual intercourse
- Back pain during menstruation
- Pain while urinating, defecating and while passing flatus while menstruating
- Abdominal pain during ovulation
- Diarrhea during menstruation and increased urination
- Fatigue

Interestingly some women experience no pain with the condition, yet it may still lead to infertility.

How does endometriosis cause infertility?

In moderate to severe cases, endometriosis can cause scarring to the fallopian tubes, causing them to get blocked. This means an egg will not be able to travel down the tube and sperm will not be able to travel up in search of an egg. Scar tissue can also envelope the ovaries, inhibiting the release of an egg. Interestingly, in many cases of endometriosis, the disease is not severe enough to cause plumbing problems, however infertility will still be present. It is thought that the inflammatory chemicals produced by a woman with endometriosis interfere with conception, implantation, and increase the risk of miscarriage.

Diagnosis and conventional treatment of endometriosis

Women who experience intense menstrual cramps, along with some of the other symptoms mentioned are usually assumed to be suffering with endometriosis. However, the only definitive way to diagnose the condition is via laparoscopy. This is a small operation performed under a general anaesthetic, where a small telescope is inserted into the abdomen through a tiny cut in the belly button. The conventional treatment of endometriosis includes non-steroidal anti-inflammatory drugs (NSAIDs) for pain relief, such as ibuprofen and naproxen. These drugs should be avoided or used with caution in women trying to conceive. Birth control pills are often recommended for women with endometriosis, as they suppress hormone production. They are obviously not appropriate in women trying to conceive and they don't address the cause of the condition anyway.

In moderate to severe endometriosis, drugs called gonadotropin releasing hormone agonists (for example Lupron [leupolide]) are given to women to put them in a temporary menopausal state. These drugs are not a permanent solution, they have terrible side effects and they can make it more difficult to conceive for women undertaking IVF. Another conventional treatment is the drug Danazol. It is a weak androgen (male hormone) and works by reducing estrogen production. Danazol has side effects and it can cause birth defects if a woman becomes pregnant. Another commonly used treatment for endometriosis is surgery to remove the endometrial deposits and scar tissue from the abdominal organs. This provides relief for a while and can help to increase a woman's chances of conception, but the tissue tends to grow back in time.

Recommended treatment for endometriosis

Endometriosis is a symptom of estrogen dominance and progesterone deficiency; therefore a cornerstone of treatment is correcting the hormone imbalance. Endometriosis also has a strong immune component; therefore improving the health of the immune system is also vitally important.

Strategies for the treatment of endometriosis:

• Try to make your diet as healthy as possible. Your hormone balance or lack thereof is greatly influenced by your day to day diet. Ensure you eat plenty of vegetables, fruit, good quality sources of protein (such as seafood, poultry, eggs - free range or organic is preferable). Keep your intake of red meat to a minimum, as it can worsen inflammation via its effect on prostaglandins, thereby worsening menstrual cramps. Minimize your intake of sugar, flour, alcohol and margarine, as all of those foods increase inflammation. Women with endometriosis don't make enough progesterone. Progesterone is a steroid hormone, meaning it is made from cholesterol. Therefore it is important to include plenty of good fats in your diet to encourage progesterone production. Good fats are found in raw nuts and seeds, oily fish (such as salmon, sardines, anchovies and mackerel), extra virgin olive oil, freshly ground flaxseeds, avocados and organic coconut oil.

- Avoid consuming cow's milk and gluten. Endometriosis displays several features of autoimmune disease, and these foods worsen inflammation and promote antibody production against your own organs and tissues. Please avoid all cow's milk and any food that is made of, or contains cow's milk. Lactose free milk is not suitable. It is not the lactose in milk that promotes immune system problems; it's the protein (casein). Gluten is found in wheat, rye, barley, oats, spelt, kamut and many processed foods. Gluten promotes auto-antibody production. All women with endometriosis need to follow our fertility diet in chapter 8 of this book.

- Correct poor liver and bowel function. The majority of women with endometriosis and other estrogen dominant conditions have sluggish liver and bowel function. Your body is constantly producing estrogen and breaking it down again and excreting it. It is your liver's job to break down estrogen after it has done its jobs in your body. Liver function can be compromised by an unhealthy diet and lifestyle; factors such as too much alcohol or sugar and not enough raw plant food put a great deal of stress on your liver. Some viruses, medication, autoimmune disease, Syndrome X (insulin resistance) and obesity also compromise liver function.

- Make sure you get enough sleep. Melatonin is a hormone made in the pineal gland of the brain that you produce when you sleep. Melatonin is available on prescription and is sometimes used by people who are suffering from jet lag and are unable to sleep, or for other causes of insomnia. Melatonin has powerful anti-inflammatory and antioxidant effects in the body; it is largely responsible for the therapeutic effects of sleep on your body. Recently a Turkish research team found that when given to rats, melatonin significantly shrank endometriosis lesions over a two month period, compared to rats who did not receive melatonin.[7] This is very promising research, but more studies need to be conducted in humans. Sleep is extremely therapeutic and you need to ensure you get enough good quality sleep each night; aim for seven to eight hours. Melatonin supplements should not be used long term.

- Minimize your exposure to environmental estrogens as much as possible. See chapter 9 for more information.
- Use natural progesterone. If the endometriosis is severe enough to interfere with your fertility, you need to use bio-identical progesterone. See page 49 for detailed information about the importance of progesterone.

Recommended nutritional supplements for endometriosis

- The most important vitamin required for progesterone production is vitamin B6. Women who experience premenstrual syndrome (PMS) are typically B6 deficient, and this worsens the condition. Symptoms such as premenstrual bloating, breast tenderness and mood disturbances all respond well to B6 supplementation. The oral contraceptive pill promotes vitamin B6 deficiency; therefore women who have taken the pill in the past are almost certainly deficient. Vitamin B6 is also required for the production of the brain chemicals (neurotransmitters) serotonin, noradrenalin, dopamine and GABA (gamma amino-butyric acid); therefore it promotes a healthy mood.

Vitamin B6 is found in small quantities in most foods, including potatoes, bananas, salmon, chicken and spinach. If you have endometriosis, problem menstrual periods or have used the pill in the past, you will not get enough through diet; a supplement is essential. Research has shown that 100 mg of vitamin B6 per day is an effective dose. If you take a vitamin B6 supplement, it is important to take a B complex supplement as well, in order to avoid developing a deficiency in other B vitamins.

• Fish oil can prevent endometriosis developing in the first place, and it is an excellent treatment for women who already have the condition. Researchers from Harvard Medical School and Boston's Brigham and Women's Hospital in the USA analyzed diet and health data from 70,709 American nurses. The total amount of fat the women consumed each day didn't affect their risk of endometriosis, but the type of fat they ate did. Women who consumed the most omega 3 fats were 22 percent less likely to be diagnosed with endometriosis within 12 years, compared with women who ate the least.

This is not surprising, as omega 3 fats are a powerful natural anti-inflammatory agent. Other research has shown that an inflammatory protein made by the immune system called Nf-Kappa B plays a key role in promoting and maintaining abnormal growth of endometrial tissue. Nf-Kappa B is a type of switch that turns on the production of a whole host of inflammatory chemicals by our cells. Chronically high blood levels of this protein are found in people who consume sugar, starch and omega 6 fat rich diets; that's most of the Western world. High levels of Nf-Kappa B are associated with several degenerative and painful diseases. The good news is that fish oil (as well as antioxidants) can suppress Nf-Kappa B production.[9]

Fish oil is an essential component of the treatment of all inflammatory diseases and immune dysfunction. Consuming oily fish in your diet, along with walnuts and freshly ground flaxseeds is very beneficial, but it is not enough if you already have endometriosis. You will need to take a fish oil supplement. A beneficial dose would be approximately 1200 mg of DHA and 1800 mg of EPA per day. You will need to find a strong, concentrated fish oil in capsule form, or use liquid fish oil to achieve that dose.

• Vitamin D has an anti-inflammatory effect in the body and is beneficial for all immune system disorders, including endometriosis. For more information on vitamin D see page 89.

- Selenium is an anti-inflammatory mineral and is necessary for women with endometriosis. See page 91 for more information on selenium.
- Vitamin E helps to reduce scar tissue and is essential for healing. Vitamin E is found in extra virgin olive oil, nuts and seeds and avocados. If you have endometriosis, you would benefit from a vitamin E supplement of 500 to 1000 IU per day. Vitamin E is best taken as mixed tocopherols.
- MSM is an organic form of sulfur; it stands for methyl sulfonyl methane. It can be taken in supplement form along with vitamin C.
- Vitamin K is found in dark green leafy vegetables and extra virgin olive oil. Deficiency of vitamin K makes it more difficult for your blood to clot; thereby promoting heavier bleeding. Including more vitamin K in your diet will help to reduce excessive menstrual bleeding.

There are several herbs that are very beneficial for correcting the hormone imbalance of endometriosis. These herbs include Vitex agnus castus, Paeonia lactiflora and Angelica sinensis. It is best to see a naturopath or herbalist, as they can recommend the ideal combination of herbs for your specific condition.

Uterine fibroids

Uterine fibroids are non-malignant tumors of the muscular wall of the uterus. They are also known as myomas and leiomyomas. It is estimated that between 30 and 50 percent of women aged 35 to 50 years have one or more uterine fibroids. They are most common in women in their late 30s up until menopause. Fibroids are sensitive to estrogen; it stimulates them to grow; especially if inadequate progesterone is produced in your body. Studies have shown that fibroids contain a greater quantity of estrogen receptors than surrounding healthy uterine tissue. When a woman reaches menopause, the lack of estrogen causes them to shrink. Hormone replacement therapy would enable fibroids to keep growing.

Symptoms of uterine fibroids

In many cases fibroids cause no symptoms and a woman may not be aware she has them. The following list describes the most common symptoms of uterine fibroids:

- Heavy menstrual bleeding and/or lengthy periods
- Menstrual cramps
- Spotting between periods
- Painful sexual intercourse (dyspareunia)
- Frequent urination if fibroids press against the bladder
- A sensation of pressure or heaviness in the back
- Backache

There are several different types of uterine fibroids, depending on their location and features; they include:

- Intramural
- Pedunculated
- Intracavitary
- Submucus
- Subserus

Uterine Fibroids

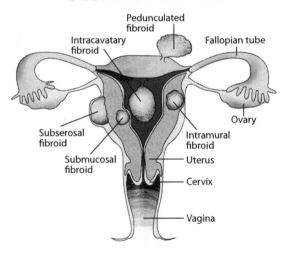

Uterine fibroids can be as small as a pea, or larger than a grapefruit. It is their size, as well as their location that determines whether they adversely affect a woman's fertility. Submucosal fibroids are most likely to interfere with fertility, mainly because they can inhibit successful implantation of an embryo. Women with intramural fibroids are also likely to have fertility problems, and they are more prone to miscarriages.[10] Intramural fibroids are the most common variety. Any type of fibroid can restrict the growth of the fetus while in the womb and this increases the risk of stillbirth (intrauterine fetal death) or premature delivery.

What causes uterine fibroids?

Estrogen fuels the growth of uterine fibroids and progesterone suppresses their growth. The same factors that promote endometriosis also promote uterine fibroids. Fibroids are the result of years of estrogen dominance and relative progesterone deficiency. Synthetic hormones found in the contraceptive pill, implant and vaginal ring, as well as the hormones in HRT (hormone replacement therapy) also fuel their growth. Environmental estrogens such as pesticides and plastic have a significantly detrimental effect on fibroids. Interestingly, research has shown that females fed soy formula in infancy are more likely to develop uterine fibroids by age 35, and so too are infants who had mothers with diabetes.[11]

Diagnosis and conventional treatment of uterine fibroids

In many cases fibroids do not cause any problems and women are not aware they have them. Fibroids can be detected during a physical examination performed by a gynecologist or general practitioner. The diagnosis needs to be confirmed with an ultrasound.

Small fibroids that are not causing any symptoms or interfering with fertility are left alone and monitored with regular ultrasounds. If fibroids are causing problems, there are a number of treatment options. Drugs can be prescribed to reduce hormone production, and this gradually shrinks the fibroids. A hysterectomy is the most common treatment for fibroids that are large and are causing heavy menstrual bleeding and discomfort; fibroids are a leading cause of hysterectomy. Clearly this is not a favorable option for women who want to have children. There are other procedures available for fibroid removal, including removing the fibroids only (during hysteroscopy), or blocking the blood supply to a fibroid (arterial embolization) so that it eventually dies. In most cases neither of those procedures is very successful, because fibroids tend to grow back, and surgically removing fibroids can weaken the uterine wall, making child bearing risky or impossible.

Often the best option for women with fibroids who want to preserve their fertility is myomectomy; this is a surgery to remove the fibroids through an incision in the abdomen. This is also the best choice for women with many fibroids (15 to 20) which are 7 cm or larger. This surgery can also be used for fibroids that are in a sensitive location, such as on top of a fallopian tube. A myomectomy is a major surgery, and requires a hospital stay of several days, and a recovery time of several weeks. Fibroids on the inside of the uterus can be removed through the vagina with a hysteroscope. This is a telescope that goes into the uterus through the vagina and cervix. Women who have this procedure can usually go home the same day and return to normal activities in around 24 hours. Another benefit of this procedure is it usually doesn't leave scars in the uterus; this is important in order to preserve fertility. This procedure is most suitable for submucosal fibroids.

Laparoscopy can be used in women with only a few fibroids that are on the outside of the uterus and that aren't larger than 6 cm. A laparoscopy is where the fibroids are removed via small incisions in the navel. After a laparoscopy women can usually leave the hospital the same day, but will need around three days to recover. The biggest drawback with laparoscopy is that the uterus must be sewn back together with multiple layers of stitches to prevent it from rupturing during pregnancy. If you wish to have this procedure, it is vital you find a highly skilled and experienced gynecologist. In most cases, women who have had fibroid surgery can attempt getting pregnant around three months later. The delivery will have to be monitored closely to make sure the uterus doesn't rupture. Some doctors strongly recommend a caesarean section instead.

Recommended nutritional treatment for uterine fibroids

The diet and supplement recommendations we give you in the following section are effective for shrinking small fibroids in the majority of cases. However, clearly it is best to try and avoid developing uterine fibroids in the first place. The problem is, when they are small and easily reversed, they often don't cause any symptoms, so women are generally unaware of their presence. It is important to remember that uterine fibroids are a consequence of estrogen dominance and progesterone deficiency. Therefore, if you have symptoms of progesterone deficiency, this needs to be corrected before it does irreparable harm to your reproductive organs. See page 49 for information about progesterone.

How to treat uterine fibroids

• Women with uterine fibroids have suffered long term progesterone deficiency. See page 49 for our recommendations on increasing your progesterone level.

• Green tea may be effective for fibroids. A study published in the American Journal of Obstetrics and Gynecology found that an extract of green tea has the ability to kill human fibroid cells in tissue cultures, and it can eradicate fibroid lesions in animals. The researchers are in the process of recruiting participants for human trials.[12]

• Reduce your exposure to environmental estrogens as much as possible. Plastic, pesticides, dioxins and several other chemicals all promote fibroid growth. See chapter 9 for more information.

• Make sure you don't have high blood insulin levels. Insulin is a growth promoting hormone, and it as well as insulin-like growth factor 1 both stimulate the growth of tumors in the body. Insulin is produced when you eat sugar, flour, grains, cereals and sugar. Therefore it is important to limit your intake of these foods.

• Have your iron level checked, as fibroids usually cause heavy bleeding which makes a woman iron deficient. Iron deficiency can inhibit ovulation.

• Take a selenium supplement, as this mineral helps to reduce the growth of benign tumors. An ideal dose is 200 micrograms of selenium per day.

• Vitamin K helps to reduce bleeding caused by fibroids. Vitamin K is found in dark green leafy vegetables and extra virgin olive oil.

Ovarian cysts

Ovarian cysts are fluid filled sacs that are common in women during their reproductive years. Most types of ovarian cysts do not cause symptoms; they are harmless and go away on their own. Every menstruating woman produces several cyst-like structures during the first half of her menstrual cycle. One "cyst" becomes the dominant follicle, which releases an egg at ovulation. If a pregnancy doesn't occur, the remaining follicle becomes the corpus luteum and then eventually breaks down and dissolves when a woman bleeds. Ovarian cysts form when this process does not develop properly and the resulting empty ovarian follicle fills with fluid and enlarges.

There are several types of ovarian cysts:

- Simple cysts, also called functional cysts. This is the most common type. These cysts are usually harmless and typically go away on their own within approximately three menstrual cycles.
- Endometrial cysts. These are sometimes called chocolate cysts because they are filled with blood. They occur when endometrial tissue attaches itself to the ovaries. If not treated promptly there is a risk these cysts can damage the ovaries and seriously impair fertility.
- Dermoid cysts. These cysts contain various types of tissue, such as hair, nails, teeth and others.
- Cystadenoma. These cysts form from cells lining the outer surface of the ovaries.

Symptoms of ovarian cysts

Ovarian cysts often cause no symptoms at all. If symptoms are present, the following may occur:

- If the cysts become very large they can cause pressure, a feeling of fullness and discomfort in the abdomen.
- Painful sexual intercourse
- A disrupted menstrual cycle and/or unusually painful menstrual periods

If a cyst becomes twisted (called torsion) this can cause intense pain; so too can a large cyst that bursts. An ultrasound or laparoscopy can diagnose ovarian cysts.

Treatment of ovarian cysts

In the case of simple cysts the usual medical approach is to wait and see. In many cases the cysts resolve themselves. Oral contraceptives are often prescribed because they inhibit ovulation and suppress production of the body's own hormones. This is not a long term solution and we do not recommend this option. If cysts are very large and causing discomfort, surgery may be required to remove them.

Most ovarian cysts will dissolve in time, with appropriate diet changes. It is vitally important for women with ovarian cysts to avoid all dairy products. Dairy products worsen cysts present anywhere in the body. A healthy diet, as described in chapter 8 should help to resolve cysts. Margarine and processed vegetable oil must be avoided. Iodine deficiency increases the risk of cysts in the ovaries, breasts and thyroid gland. Many women are iodine deficient. We recommend an iodine intake of between 160 and 350 mcg in supplement form per day. Women with thyroid dysfunction are at increased risk of ovarian cysts. Treating the thyroid problem with nutritional medicine usually resolves ovarian cysts as well.

Selenium and vitamin D are also beneficial for helping to shrink ovarian cysts. You can find these nutrients combined in supplement form called Thyroid Health Capsules. If you have questions about nutrients required for overcoming ovarian cysts, please phone Dr Cabot's Health Advisory Line in Australia on 02 4655 8855 or the United States of America on 623 334 3232 or email contact@weightcontroldoctor.com.

Polycystic Ovarian Syndrome (PCOS)

Polycystic ovarian syndrome is the most common hormonal disorder affecting women in their reproductive life; a Melbourne study conducted in 2005 found that it affects 12 percent of Australian women.[13] The incidence is similar in all Western nations, including the USA. Polycystic ovarian syndrome is the most common hormonal disorder causing female infertility.[14]

Symptoms of Polycystic Ovarian Syndrome

As the name suggests, women with PCOS have cysts on their ovaries. In most cases the cysts are tiny; they were ovarian follicles that failed to develop fully. Normal healthy women produce multiple ovarian follicles each month that contain developing eggs. As ovulation approaches, one of these follicles matures fully and releases a ripe egg; that is ovulation. The rest of the follicles dissolve and are reabsorbed by the ovary. In the case of PCOS, the follicles do not form properly. Therefore an ultrasound of the ovaries will reveal multiple small under-developed follicles. Because the follicles don't develop fully, ovulation does not occur. Obviously these women have a great deal of trouble falling pregnant because with no egg, fertilization is impossible.

An ultrasound is not enough to diagnose PCOS. It is a hormonal disorder and this disruption in hormones produces a range of symptoms. The following list describes the most common symptoms of PCOS. You may have some or all of these symptoms.

Characteristics of polycystic ovarian syndrome

- Obesity, particularly in the abdominal region
- Hirsutism (excessive hair growth, particularly on the face, chest and abdomen)
- Irregular or absent menstruation
- Anovulation (lack of ovulation)
- Insulin resistance (syndrome X), characterized by high blood fasting insulin levels and other indicators.
- Progesterone deficiency
- PMS, painful and heavy menstrual periods. These symptoms may be present and are due to progesterone deficiency.
- Polycystic ovaries (seen on ultrasound)
- Acne, especially around the jaw line, chest and back
- Greasy skin
- Sometimes the hormone prolactin is elevated
- Most women with PCOS are deficient in vitamin D and iodine.
- Scalp hair loss in the male pattern (front and sides)

Women with PCOS produce too much luteinizing hormone (LH); typically they have twice as much LH as FSH (follicle stimulating hormone) on a blood test. This does not allow ovarian follicles to develop properly and disrupts normal ovulation. The ovaries produce too high quantities of male hormones (androgens), such as testosterone.

The underlying hormone imbalance in PCOS is insulin resistance. Women with this condition produce too much insulin and their body does not respond to it properly. It is insulin that triggers the hormone abnormalities seen in PCOS and insulin triggers the ovaries to produce testosterone.

Women with PCOS often have a family history of type 2 diabetes or obesity, particularly apple shaped obesity (abdominal obesity). People with these conditions usually over produce insulin in response to carbohydrate in their diet. Women with PCOS do not cope well with "normal" or common levels of carbohydrate in their diet. A low carbohydrate diet is the most essential component of the treatment of PCOS.

Because women with PCOS do not ovulate, or don't ovulate regularly, they cannot manufacture progesterone. Therefore they can experience the symptoms of progesterone deficiency listed on page 50. Progesterone deficiency also increases the risk of miscarriage, endometrial cancer (cancer of the lining of the uterus) and breast cancer. The lack of progesterone causes changes in the lining of the uterus (endometrium) which make implantation of an embryo more difficult. This further complicates a woman's chances of becoming pregnant.

Because they are insulin resistant, women with PCOS are at increased risk of type 2 diabetes, heart attacks and strokes. They have a greater risk of gestational diabetes (diabetes in pregnancy) and miscarriage. Women with PCOS have a high failure rate with IVF. They are more prone to having an adverse reaction from the hormones used; that is they are more prone to ovarian hyperstimulation. They also have poorer quality eggs and an increased risk of miscarriage.[15]

Diagnosis of PCOS

Blood tests for the following are required to confirm the diagnosis:

- Free androgen index, total testosterone and free testosterone. These are male hormones and they are typically elevated. The normal reference ranges for these hormones are stated in chapter 10.

- SHBG (sex hormone binding globulin). This is a protein made in the liver that binds to estrogen and testosterone and carries them around the bloodstream. The high blood insulin levels in women with PCOS inhibit the liver's production of SHBG. Consequently women have higher levels of free testosterone in their bloodstream. This is what causes most of the symptoms of PCOS.
- Dehydroepiandrosterone (DHEA). This a hormone made predominantly in the adrenal glands. It is often elevated and contributes to the symptoms of excess androgens (male hormones).
- Fasting blood insulin. This is elevated in the majority of cases and is a result of insulin resistance. A fasting insulin level of 10 U/L or higher indicates insulin resistance.
- Fasting blood glucose and/or glucose tolerance test with insulin. This is one indicator of insulin resistance and is also required because women with PCOS are at increased risk of type 2 diabetes.
- Luteinizing hormone (LH). Typically LH is elevated and is usually twice as high as FSH (follicle stimulating hormone).
- Follicle stimulating hormone (FSH). This is required in order to check the ovaries' capacity to produce estrogen.
- Prolactin. This hormone is made by the pituitary gland in the brain. It is elevated in approximately 25 percent of PCOS patients. Prolactin is covered in detail later in this chapter.
- Serum vitamin D test. Many PCOS patients are vitamin D deficient and deficiency will worsen anovulation.
- Urinary iodine test. Iodine deficiency is common in these patients.

Testing for insulin resistance (syndrome X)

We have said that the underlying cause of PCOS is insulin resistance. So how do you know if you have insulin resistance? An official diagnosis can be made based on the following five criteria. If you can tick at least three of the boxes, you officially have insulin resistance:

1. *Fasting blood glucose of 99mg/dL (5.5 mmol/L) or higher.*
2. *Waist circumference greater than 33 inches (85cm) in women.*

3. *Fasting triglycerides of 149 mg/dL (1.69 mmol/L) or higher.*
4. *Fasting HDL cholesterol ("good cholesterol") less than 38.6 mg/dL (1 mmol/L)*
5. *Blood pressure greater than 130/85 mmHg*

It is also beneficial to have a fasting insulin blood test or a two hour glucose tolerance test with insulin. These tests are useful for diagnosing insulin resistance, even though they are not used in official diagnostic criteria.

Nearly every woman with PCOS meets at least three of the diagnostic criteria for insulin resistance, and in fact nearly every person in Western society fits the bill. Insulin resistance is caused by eating more carbohydrate than your body was designed to eat. Our bodies were not designed to eat much carbohydrate at all. For the majority of human history we survived as hunters and gatherers, living off vegetables, fruit, animal meat, fish, poultry, eggs, nuts and seeds. We simply did not have the machinery available to process grains and turn them into flour. Today the average person's diet is based on grains, cereals, starches and sugar. Naturally this has health consequences. You do not need to be overweight to have insulin resistance. Your health will suffer if you eat too much carbohydrate whether you are overweight or not.

Orthodox medical treatment of polycystic ovarian syndrome

The following medications are typically used to manage PCOS:

The oral contraceptive pill (OCP)

This is commonly given to women to enable them to have a regular menstrual bleed and give the appearance of regulating their menstrual cycle. Of course the pill does not fix the underlying condition and it is not an appropriate treatment for women wishing to conceive. The pill helps to prevent overgrowth of the uterine lining (endometrium) associated with progesterone deficiency, but prescribed natural progesterone can achieve the same benefits. The pill can reduce the symptoms of excess male hormones, such as acne, scalp hair loss and facial hair, however symptoms return once the pill is stopped. Oral contraceptives that contain cyproterone acetate (eg. Brenda-35 ED and Diane-35 ED) are most commonly used, but they increase the risk of blood clots and high cholesterol. Most women with PCOS are already at increased risk of these conditions. The oral contraceptive pill is a completely ineffective way to manage PCOS, and in fact some forms of the pill are believed to cause the condition in the first place.

Anti male hormone medication

These drugs work by reducing the body's production of androgens (male hormones), interfering with the action of androgens, and/or increasing the production of sex hormone binding globulin (SHBG). These drugs are usually very effective at reducing the symptoms of excess male hormones (such as facial hair, scalp hair loss and acne). These drugs are not useful for women wishing to get pregnant, as they would cause severe birth defects. Examples of medications in this category are Androcur (cyproterone acetate) and Aldactone (spironolactone).

Metformin

This is a drug used for type 2 diabetes and insulin resistance. Metformin acts to reduce the liver's production of glucose, reduce the intestinal absorption of glucose and improve insulin sensitivity. Because it addresses the cause of PCOS (insulin resistance), it does offer benefits and can help women to ovulate more regularly. However Metformin should not be used in pregnancy and it depletes the body of vitamin B12.

Recommendations for the treatment of polycystic ovarian syndrome

Polycystic ovarian syndrome responds extremely well to diet and lifestyle changes, as well as the use of bio-identical progesterone. The underlying cause of PCOS is insulin resistance; therefore it must be corrected to overcome the condition. Nutritional deficiencies and other hormonal problems are sometimes present, and they too must be corrected. We recommend the following for PCOS:

- A low carbohydrate diet is essential. Women with PCOS cannot cope with common levels of carbohydrate in their diet. A low carbohydrate diet will lower blood insulin levels and that will greatly reduce the ovaries' production of male hormones. A low carbohydrate diet will also enable weight loss from the abdominal region and upper body, and that too will enable a reduction in male hormone levels. Losing weight, lowering your insulin level and eating less carbohydrate are the most effective natural ways to start ovulating regularly.

Even slim women with PCOS must avoid sugar and high glycemic index carbohydrates, as research has shown these foods both increase testosterone levels, and increase the body's sensitivity to the testosterone already present. Therefore sugar, bread, pasta, rice, breakfast cereals, potatoes and all foods containing grains and flour need to be strictly limited or avoided. See the section that follows for our low carbohydrate diet guidelines. If you find weight loss extremely difficult, you may need to reduce your carbohydrate intake to approximately 30 grams per day, in order to get your body to burn fat. This should be done under the supervision of a naturopath or nutritionist.

- Avoid damaged vegetable fats. These are found in margarine and most vegetable oil sold for cooking, as well as processed foods that list vegetable oil in the ingredients list. These fats worsen insulin resistance and they promote weight gain. They can also inhibit you from ovulating. Beneficial fats to include in your diet are extra virgin olive oil, cold pressed macadamia nut oil, organic coconut oil and small amounts of ghee.
- Exercise is essential. Exercise reverses insulin resistance because it makes your muscle cells more sensitive to insulin. Exercise will also help you lose weight. A combination of aerobic exercise that makes you huff and puff, and muscle strengthening exercises is ideal.
- Have a blood test for your thyroid function. Many women with PCOS also have an under active thyroid gland and this makes weight loss and conception much more difficult. Research has shown that women with PCOS have a higher prevalence of autoimmune thyroid disease.[16] This may be because these women are progesterone deficient, and progesterone has a beneficial anti-inflammatory effect on the immune system.
- Have a blood test for vitamin D. Vitamin D deficiency aggravates hormone disorders and many Australian women are deficient. Your blood vitamin D level should be between

100 and 150 nmol/L (40 to 60 ng/mL).
- Have a urine test for iodine. Iodine deficiency is extremely common and deficiency of this mineral increases the risk of cysts in the ovaries, breasts and thyroid gland. You are considered to have sufficient iodine in your body if your urine level is above 100 micrograms per liter.
- Avoid using the birth control pill, as it may worsen insulin resistance.
- Increase your intake of magnesium and chromium. Both of these minerals are essential for helping to make your cells more sensitive to insulin; thus they help to reverse insulin resistance. They will reduce hunger and cravings and make a low carbohydrate diet much easier to stick to. Deficiencies of these minerals are very common, but blood tests are not an accurate way to determine this. An ideal daily dose of magnesium is 400 mg; it is easier to achieve this dose with a magnesium supplement in powder form. An ideal dose of chromium is 200 mcg per day. It is not possible to obtain those quantities through your diet; supplements are required.
- The herbs Gymnema sylvestre and bitter melon help to improve insulin sensitivity as well as reducing carbohydrate cravings.
- Try to minimize stress. This is easier said than done, considering that infertility itself is a very stressful condition. Unfortunately stress is a big driver of PCOS, especially in normal weight and slim women. Magnesium, B vitamins and vitamin C all help the adrenal glands to recuperate from long term stress. Adequate sleep and rest are also essential for helping the body to recover from stress.
- Bio-identical progesterone cream is necessary. This will help to suppress LH (luteinizing hormone) production by the pituitary gland, thus allowing ovulation to occur. Progesterone helps to reset the pituitary gland, thus restoring a regular monthly bleed. See page 49 for more information about progesterone.

Low carbohydrate diet guidelines

This is the eating plan we recommend for women with polycystic ovarian syndrome, type 2 diabetics and anyone who needs to lose weight. Our books *Can't Lose Weight?*

Unlock the Secrets that keep you Fat and *Diabetes Type 2: You can reverse it* both contain recipes and meal plans for a low carbohydrate diet. This is a strict diet, but it is designed to achieve a purpose. You will not have to avoid carbohydrate rich foods so drastically forever.

Avoid

GRAINS – wheat, rye, oats, barley, corn, rice, spelt, kamut, flour, bread, cereal, pasta, noodles, pastry, crackers.

POTATOES, BANANAS

SUGAR, HONEY, JAM, GOLDEN SYRUP

ALL FOODS CONTAINING SUGAR – sweets, chocolate, ice-cream, sweet yoghurt

MARGARINE

Good Foods

SALADS – dress with extra virgin olive oil, macadamia oil, vinegar, lemon or lime juice, mustard.

COOKED VEGETABLES except potatoes and corn

SEAFOOD, POULTRY, EGGS, RED MEAT

FRUIT – limit of 2 pieces per day. No dried fruit or fruit juice.

LEGUMES – eg. Beans, peas, lentils, chickpeas, hummus

NUTS AND SEEDS – not roasted or salted though

Canned coconut milk, almond milk, unsweetened soy milk.

Suggested Menu

Breakfast: Poached, boiled or scrambled eggs with mushrooms, tomato, asparagus, spinach.

Omelette containing some left over vegetables from last night's dinner

Protein Powder smoothie containing fruit

Dinner left overs – such as soup on a cold winter morning

Lunch: Canned fish with salad

Left over chicken or roast meat with salad

Rissoles with salad or cooked vegetables

Left over stew or curry from dinner

Chicken Caesar salad without croutons

Greek salad combined with canned fish or chicken

Go to a sandwich bar and get the sandwich filling (chicken, fish, eggs, salad) in a box. You don't have to buy a sandwich; just buy the filling.

Dinner: Baked or grilled fish with salad

Baked dinner without potatoes (use pumpkin, carrot, green beans, onion, squash, beetroot, sweet potato).

Roast chicken with salad or cooked vegetables

Stew, curry, casserole, stir fry or goulash without rice, pasta, noodles or potatoes.

Bolognaise served over steamed vegetables.

Snacks: Fruit with raw nuts and seeds

Protein powder smoothie

Hummus with vegetable sticks

Celery with nut butter

Not all women with PCOS are overweight!

The vast majority of women with PCOS are overweight, but some are not. Normal weight and slim women can be diagnosed with PCOS. They may have high or normal blood levels of testosterone, and normal insulin levels. However, even though these women are not overweight, some research has shown they still overproduce insulin in response to carbohydrate ingestion. In addition, although they appear slim, these women often have higher than desirable levels of visceral fat (meaning fat within and around the abdominal organs).

Therefore, even if you are slim, you still need to follow a low carbohydrate diet. Stress and poor diet seem to be major contributing factors to PCOS in normal weight women. It is also thought that the predisposition to develop PCOS occurs when a woman is a fetus in her mother's uterus. Exposure to high levels of testosterone in-utero greatly increases a woman's risk of developing PCOS.

Ovarian drilling: A procedure best avoided

Ovarian drilling is a procedure sometimes used on PCOS patients to help them achieve regular menstrual cycles and reduce their level of testosterone. It's a terrible sounding name, but in reality it is a minimally invasive laparoscopic procedure. A tiny camera attached to a thin telescope is inserted into a small incision below the belly button. During the procedure, very small holes are made in the ovaries, which reduce the ability of the ovaries to manufacture testosterone. Women with PCOS typically have ovaries that have a thicker outer surface than normal. Ovarian drilling breaks through the thick outer surface. The procedure does help many women to achieve regular menstrual periods, and it reduces testosterone levels, thus reducing many of the symptoms of PCOS. However, the benefits are usually short lived and the full gamut of PCOS symptoms usually returns in time. If you are able to fall pregnant after ovarian drilling, you are less likely to have twins or triplets compared to women with PCOS taking the fertility drug clomiphene.

Ovarian drilling has significant disadvantages and risks. The procedure may cause injury to the intestines, bladder, ureters or blood vessels. This is the case with any laparoscopic procedure. There is a minor risk of bleeding, infection or a reaction to the anaesthetic. The biggest risk associated with ovarian drilling is experiencing an early menopause. Women who have this procedure performed are likely to enter menopause sooner than women who haven't had it done. This means they may have fewer fertile years in which to try and conceive. Ovarian drilling also increases the risk that a woman will develop autoimmune ovarian failure. It increases the likelihood that a woman will produce antibodies against her own ovaries and go on to develop premature ovarian failure.[17] This condition is covered in more detail in chapter 5

Case study: polycystic ovarian syndrome

When Meredith arrived at my clinic she had a thick folder of paperwork detailing all the infertility tests she had performed. Meredith was 35 and as far as the tests showed, polycystic ovarian syndrome was the main cause of her infertility. Meredith was significantly overweight and had suffered with very irregular menstrual periods for the last five years.

When Meredith did get a period, it was extremely heavy and painful. Blood tests showed that Meredith had significant insulin resistance and if she wasn't careful, she was well on her way to type 2 diabetes. Unfortunately Meredith loved carbohydrate rich foods. She ate lots of bread, toast, pasta, rice, breakfast cereals, biscuits and chocolate each day. She also drank three cups of tea each day and had four teaspoons of sugar in each one! Meredith was always hungry; she confessed to thinking about food all day. No wonder; all these carbohydrate rich foods raise blood insulin levels and would make anyone ravenous. Meredith told me that she had been to see a dietician but she could not follow the diet. She said she wants to fall pregnant but would not be making any changes to her diet! I had my work cut out for me.

Somehow I managed to convince Meredith that what she was eating each day was the greatest determinant of her hormone levels. By lowering her carbohydrate intake, she would reduce her insulin level, reduce her risk of diabetes, normalize her menstrual cycle and ovulate regularly. Along with the low carbohydrate diet, I put Meredith on Magnesium Ultra Potent powder (to help with stress and insulin resistance) and Glycemic Balance capsules (to reduce her cravings for carbohydrate). Meredith's blood test showed her to be severely vitamin D deficient; therefore I gave her a supplement. Meredith also began using a progesterone cream each evening.

I saw Meredith four weeks later and she was already a changed woman. She had adhered strictly to the low carbohydrate diet and took all her supplements as directed. Meredith had lost six kilos in that time and was absolutely thrilled. The first two weeks of the diet were tough, but after that time Meredith was amazed at how easy the meal plan was to stick to. Because she stopped eating grains, sugar and starches, her appetite had drastically declined. She commented how nice it was to not be thinking about food all day. She also told me how much calmer she felt and that minor stress at work was no longer getting her down.

I saw Meredith again two months later and she was still losing weight at a steady pace and still enjoying the diet. A blood test revealed that Meredith was iron deficient; therefore I started her on an iron supplement. I also gave her a fish oil supplement at that time. She had started menstruating regularly and her period pain was greatly reduced.

Meredith's blood test results showed dramatic improvements at the six month mark. Unfortunately she suffered some personal stress at that time and lost motivation with her diet. She regained seven kilos of the 35 kilos she had lost since first seeing me. She managed to get back on track, and stepped up her exercise and four months after that she fell pregnant and had a healthy baby girl. Meredith's case of PCOS was quite long standing, and it often takes six months to a year of consistent dietary changes in order to reverse the condition and achieve pregnancy. Meredith will always have the tendency towards PCOS, but maintaining a low carbohydrate eating plan and exercising regularly can help to keep it at bay.

Elevated Prolactin
Hyperprolactinemia

Prolactin is a hormone made by the anterior pituitary gland in the brain. The function of prolactin is to enhance breast development during pregnancy, and to induce lactation. However all women and men make low levels of this hormone continually. Prolactin can be measured in a blood test and it needs to be done in a fasting state. The normal range for women is 2 - 29 ng/mL(85 - 500 mIU/L). In men the normal range is 2 - 18 ng/mL (150 – 500 mIU/L).

Elevated prolactin can cause anovulation (lack of ovulation), infrequent menstrual periods, a shortened luteal phase or a loss of menstruation altogether. The fact that prolactin usually inhibits ovulation explains why most women cannot fall pregnant while breast feeding.

Depending on how high the prolactin level is, women may experience symptoms of a milky discharge from the breasts. High levels of prolactin in the blood usually cause a loss of libido and in men they can cause erectile dysfunction.

Cause of excess prolactin production

The following factors may predispose a woman to hyperprolactinemia:

- Stress
- Some medication, particularly anti-depressants, opiates, cimetidine (used to suppress stomach acid), metoclopramide (used for nausea and vomiting), some anti-psychotic drugs and some antihistamines
- A small tumor in the pituitary gland of the brain
- Other pituitary or hypothalamic tumors interfering with dopamine production
- Women with polycystic ovarian syndrome often have mildly raised prolactin
- An under active thyroid gland
- Strenuous exercise can temporarily raise prolactin.

Because stress can cause elevated prolactin, if you do have a slightly high reading on a blood test, it is important to have it rechecked, just in case stress caused a temporary elevation. A pituitary tumor causing excess prolactin secretion is called a prolactinoma. These tumors are usually benign (non-cancerous) and are mostly very small (known as a micro-adenoma). A CT scan or MRI can detect these tumors. An MRI is preferable because it does not expose the body to radiation.

The brain chemical dopamine is responsible for suppressing excess prolactin production; therefore anything that interferes with dopamine production can allow prolactin levels to escalate. Several of the medications listed previously cause hyperprolactinemia because they reduce dopamine production. Sometimes prolactin levels only rise at night time and this makes it difficult to detect on a blood test. Women with elevated prolactin at night commonly experience breast tenderness in the week or so before a menstrual period.

Treatment of hyperprolactinemia

If a pituitary tumor is producing excess prolactin, a prescription medication called bromocriptine (Parlodel or Cycloset) is commonly used. This drug lowers prolactin levels, shrinks the pituitary tumor and restores regular ovulation and menstruation. It is best to start with a small dose of bromocriptine, as it can cause nausea and dizziness. The dose can be increased gradually until the prolactin level is normalized. Another medication called Cabergoline can also be used for the same purpose but it is not suitable for women wishing to become pregnant.

Fortunately it is usually possible to reduce excess prolactin just with dietary changes, natural progesterone and herbal medicine. We have found that eliminating all dairy products from the diet is very important for women with hyperprolactinemia. The hormones found in dairy products may stimulate the pituitary gland to manufacture excess prolactin. Therefore all cow, goat and sheep milk should be avoided, along with foods that contain milk. It is also important to increase the quantity of antioxidants in your diet, through fresh vegetables, fruit and vegetable juices.

The herbs licorice (Glycyrrhiza glabra) and peony (Paeonia lactiflora) have demonstrated an ability to lower prolactin levels nearly as well as bromocriptine, but with no side effects.[18] The herb Vitex agnus-castus is excellent for lowering prolactin because it has a dopaminergic effect; meaning it stimulates dopamine release. Increased dopamine then inhibits prolactin secretion. Vitex is effective for lowering elevated prolactin in both men and women. In women Vitex is also highly effective for premenstrual mastalgia (breast pain) and premenstrual syndrome (PMS). It is best to consult a naturopath of herbalist who will be able to prescribe the most appropriate herbs for you, at an effective dose.

Case study: High prolactin

Kara was a delightful 29 year old woman who had been diagnosed at the age of 23 with a tiny tumor on her pituitary gland. This was so tiny it could only be seen on an MRI scan of her pituitary gland and was called a micro-adenoma. This tumor secreted excessive amounts of the hormone prolactin and her blood levels of prolactin were elevated measuring 1020 mIU/L.

This tumor was so tiny that it did not produce any troubling symptoms such as headaches or visual disturbances and she only knew it was there when her menstrual periods ceased to come on a regular monthly basis and she had some breast milk from her nipples if she squeezed them. This is when her doctor decided to investigate her by checking her blood hormone levels; these were all normal except for raised prolactin.

Kara wanted her periods to come every month so her doctor gave her a drug called Kripton to lower prolactin levels. This did the trick and after 3 months her prolactin levels were normal and her periods came back. High prolactin levels stimulate the breasts to produce milk and this is normal in the postnatal period when women are breast feeding their babies. High prolactin levels suppress ovulation in the ovaries so that no progesterone is produced and thus menstrual bleeding ceases. Without ovulation infertility occurs.

What caused Kara's pituitary gland to over produce prolactin when she was 23 years old? The only obvious causes were that she was overweight with a BMI of 32 and she was highly stressed. Her diet at this time was very high in sweet foods high in carbohydrate and very high in dairy products. Cow's milk contains cow's prolactin and this can stimulate the pituitary production of prolactin. Obviously dietary factors were significant in Kara's case. Other causes of high prolactin are inadequate progesterone levels, which is a very common problem in women today.

Once Kara got to the age of 29 she wanted to have children but she did not want to have to be taking drugs to lower prolactin whilst trying to conceive. She wanted to lower her prolactin levels naturally without any drugs and to conceive naturally.

I gave her the following program –

- A low carbohydrate and dairy free diet
- An exercise program to get her weight down into the healthy range
- Natural progesterone cream in a dose of 100mg daily which would restore a regular monthly menstrual cycle and

should re-set her pituitary gland to regulate natural and spontaneous ovulation from her ovaries
* *Supplements of fish oil, iodine, selenium and zinc to help her ovaries sustain healthy eggs which ovulated and produced plentiful amounts of progesterone.*

After 4 months on the above program, I stopped Kara's medication and she continued to ovulate and have regular menstruation. After another 3 months I rechecked her blood prolactin levels and they were normal at 400 mIU/L.

Three months later Kara missed her periods and felt a little bloated and nauseated – guess what? Her pregnancy test was positive; she was thrilled as she had achieved her goal of conceiving without drugs!

I advised Kara to continue with her progesterone cream for the first four months of her pregnancy to reduce the risk of early miscarriage.

The Importance of Progesterone in Achieving and Maintaining Pregnancy

Progesterone has an enormous impact on your fertility, on your menstrual cycle and on your overall state of health. The main female sex hormones are estrogen and progesterone. Progesterone is required in order to balance the effects of estrogen in your body. Estrogen causes the cells lining your uterus to grow and divide, whereas progesterone inhibits this growth. Estrogen can be described as a fertilizer, and progesterone as a lawn mower. Progesterone is often referred to as the fertility hormone, and its name comes from the words pro gestation. This is because progesterone plays three vitally important roles in pregnancy:

* Progesterone maintains and prepares the lining of your uterus (endometrium), in preparation for the arrival and implantation of a fertilized egg.
* After implantation, progesterone is necessary for maintaining the pregnancy and reducing the risk of miscarriage.
* Progesterone has immune enhancing effects and can reduce the risk of inflammation and immune generated infertility or miscarriage.

During the first half of your menstrual cycle (follicular phase), your endometrial lining is relatively thin. Just before ovulation, it starts to thicken. Your endometrium continues to thicken after ovulation. If you do not become pregnant, your endometrial lining will be shed and you will have a menstrual bleed. If you do become pregnant, your endometrial lining remains thick, in anticipation of the arrival of an embryo. The thickness of your endometrial lining throughout your menstrual cycle is largely determined by the amount of progesterone in your body.

Progesterone is produced after ovulation, by the sac left behind after an egg is released. The empty sac is known as the corpus luteum. When you do become pregnant, the corpus luteum will continue making progesterone for approximately the first eight weeks of pregnancy. After that time, the placenta has formed and it takes over progesterone production. The placenta produces phenomenally high levels of progesterone, which increase as the pregnancy progresses. In a normal menstrual cycle, you will only produce progesterone if you have ovulated. Unfortunately, ovulation disorders are extremely common and are a leading cause of female infertility. Many women ovulate irregularly or not at all. This is most common in women with polycystic ovarian syndrome, insulin resistance, obesity, or in under weight women.

Estrogen dominance is a common cause of infertility

Progesterone deficiency is an extremely common phenomenon in today's world for a number of reasons. When a woman does not produce enough progesterone to counterbalance the effects of estrogen, we say she has a relative progesterone deficiency and therefore suffers with estrogen dominance.

Symptoms of progesterone deficiency include:

- Heavy periods
- Painful periods. Normal period pain does not last for more than 24 hours
- Infrequent periods or irregular periods
- Endometriosis
- Uterine fibroids
- Adenomyosis – thickening of the uterine muscle

- Endometrial hyperplasia (excessively thick endometrium) and polyps
- Premenstrual syndrome (PMS)
- Polycystic ovarian syndrome (PCOS)
- Postnatal depression
- Premenstrual moodiness
- Scalp hair loss or thinning
- Breast pain and/or lumpy breasts
- Insomnia in the week before menstruation and during the peri-menopause
- Worsening of autoimmune disease in women
- Worsening of thyroid problems in women
- Persistently elevated prolactin levels

The following factors can cause or contribute to estrogen dominance and progesterone deficiency:

- Anovulation (lack of ovulation). Most commonly caused by a high carbohydrate diet, nutrient deficiencies, excessive exercise, ageing or stress.
- Excess body weight
- Thyroid problems – under or overactive
- Exposure to environmental estrogens (xeno-estrogens) in pesticides, plastic, diet and pollution.
- History of use of synthetic estrogens, such as in birth control pills.
- Stress, which can cause progesterone to be converted to the stress hormone cortisol.
- Poor bowel function and a sluggish liver, which impair your body's ability to excrete estrogen.
- Excess alcohol consumption, which impairs estrogen excretion
- Poor diet, especially diets high in sugar and trans fatty acids (processed vegetable oil)

Estrogen dominance has been strongly linked with a number of adverse health outcomes. Correcting a progesterone deficiency is critical for overcoming infertility. You can modify your diet and lifestyle in various ways to help your body produce progesterone. This is important and will help to improve your fertility. However, in the vast majority of cases of infertility, we recommend you use a natural progesterone supplement. This will be explained further along in this chapter.

Help your body to produce more progesterone

- Ensure your diet is as healthy as possible. Your hormone levels are greatly influenced by the food you eat each day. Ensure you consume plenty of vegetables and fruit and protein (such as seafood, poultry, eggs) and red meat if you wish. Free range or organic is preferable. Progesterone is a steroid hormone, meaning it is made of fat; therefore it is important to include plenty of good fats in your diet if you want to improve progesterone production. Good fats are found in raw nuts and seeds, oily fish (such as salmon, sardines, mackerel and anchovies), extra virgin olive oil, avocados, freshly ground flaxseeds, chia seeds and organic coconut oil.
- Ensure that you are ovulating. The most common reason women fail to ovulate is because they have high blood insulin levels due to consuming too much carbohydrate; this often results in polycystic ovarian syndrome.
- Try to minimize stress and get 8 hours of sleep every night. Stress has the ability to disrupt hormone production by the pituitary gland in your brain, potentially disrupting your menstrual cycle and inhibiting ovulation. Women who are chronically stressed convert too much of their progesterone into cortisol. Regular exercise reduces stress and improves circulation to the ovaries.
- Include phyto-estrogens in your diet. Phyto-estrogens are plant estrogens. They are very weak estrogens and can have a balancing effect on hormones in your body. Including more phyto-estrogens in your diet can counteract some of the effects of the more powerful estrogens your own body makes. Phyto-estrogens are abundantly found in all plant foods; particularly legumes, nuts, seeds, vegetables and fruit. Grind whole flaxseeds into a fine powder and store this in the fridge; consume one to two tablespoons daily. Whole ground flaxseeds contain powerful phyto-estrogens called lignans. They not only improve fertility, they also reduce your risk of many types of cancer.
- Ensure your body excretes estrogen adequately. Your body is continually making estrogen, breaking it down and trying

to excrete it. The health of your bowels and liver determines how well you eliminate estrogen from your body.

Maintaining a healthy liver

Estrogen is broken down in your liver; some of it leaves your body in bowel movements and some is excreted in your urine. The better these organs of elimination work, the more efficiently you will be excreting estrogen. The most common cause of compromised liver function is fatty liver disease, also known as non-alcoholic steatorrhoeic hepatosis (NASH). Other factors that compromise liver function include excess alcohol intake, allergies, overgrowth of bad bowel bacteria, certain autoimmune diseases, some viruses and some medication.

You can improve the health of your liver by following a liver friendly diet. Make sure you eat at least five serves of vegetables each day. You should also eat two serves of fruit each day, and not more than that if you are overweight, diabetic or have polycystic ovarian syndrome. Please consume some vegetables raw, as in salads. Include some vegetables that are high in the mineral sulfur, as sulfur improves detoxification of estrogen in the liver. Vegetables high in sulfur include onions, leeks, garlic, cabbage, broccoli, Brussels sprouts, kale, bok choy and cauliflower. Supplements of selenium also improve liver detoxification.

You also need to eat adequate protein each day. Your liver needs the amino acids (building blocks of protein) to carry out phase one and two detoxification. Good fats are important for the liver also because they are anti-inflammatory and support the liver cell membranes.

The leading cause of fatty liver disease is a diet too high in sugar and refined carbohydrate. That means too much bread, pasta, potatoes, rice, breakfast cereals and foods containing flour or sugar. If you want to maintain good liver function it is essential you restrict your intake of these foods, particularly if you are the type of person who gains weight around their abdominal area. When carbohydrate rich foods are eaten in excess, the liver converts them into fat, promoting the development of a fatty liver and weight gain. See my book *Fatty Liver you can Reverse it* for more information.

Maintaining healthy bowels

Once estrogen is broken down in your liver, much of it is secreted into bile. Bile enters your small intestine and then the estrogen metabolites are excreted in bowel movements. If you are prone to constipation you will not be excreting estrogen adequately. Women with constipation are much more prone to experiencing symptoms of estrogen dominance.

The average person eats at least three times a day, therefore ideally you would be having between one and three bowel movements each day. If stool is allowed to remain in your colon longer, bacteria naturally present there, convert the estrogen into a more harmful form, which is absorbed into your bloodstream.

Avoiding constipation is important, but so is maintaining high levels of good bacteria in your intestines. Taking a probiotic supplement can help you to achieve regular bowel habits and will reduce the level of toxic estrogen metabolites in your body.

Here are some tips to help keep your bowels healthy:

- Drink approximately two liters of water each day. This will soften your stool and allow it to pass more easily. Avoid consuming too much tea, as the tannins in it can be constipating.
- Be more active. Exercise stimulates peristalsis (intestinal contractions).
- Ensure your diet is high in fiber rich food such as vegetables, fruit, raw nuts and seeds.
- Freshly ground flaxseeds (linseeds) are extremely high in fiber and are an excellent natural laxative. Try to consume one or two tablespoons of flaxseed meal each day if you are prone to constipation.
- When you wake, drink a cup of warm water with the juice of half a lemon. The lemon will stimulate the production of bile, which is your body's own natural laxative. The warm water will relax your bowel muscles.
- Magnesium relaxes the nerves and muscles of your bowels and is excellent for people who are prone to constipation when stressed or anxious. Magnesium powder is a more powerful laxative than magnesium tablets.

- Answer the call of nature. Try not to delay a bowel movement when you need to go.
- Avoid all laxatives that contain the herbs senna or cascara. They are habit forming and will make constipation worse in the long run.
- Avoid taking antacids and medication that blocks the production of stomach acid.
- Minimize your use of antibiotic drugs.
- In some people a food allergy or intolerance is responsible for irritable bowel syndrome and constipation. Common culprits include gluten, dairy products, soy and nuts. It is best to consult a naturopath who can help you identify problematic foods.
- Minimize your exposure to environmental estrogens. Some environmental estrogens are up to 1000 times more potent than the estrogen made in your own body. They can have a powerfully disruptive effect on your hormone levels. See chapter 9 for information on environmental estrogens.
- Certain herbs can help to increase your body's production of progesterone. It is best that you consult a naturopath if you wish to use herbs, as many herbs are not suitable for use during pregnancy.

Bioidentical progesterone supplementation

If you are struggling with infertility, it is probably necessary for you to use a progesterone supplement, as well as following the diet and lifestyle recommendations just made. Inadequate progesterone production during pregnancy can impair implantation of the embryo in your endometrium and it can increase the risk of miscarriage. Progesterone deficiency during early pregnancy can increase the risk of your immune system rejecting the embryo.

Progesterone has the following immune system benefits during pregnancy:

- Reduces inflammation that can lead to scarring and damage to the placenta.
- Reduces the ability of natural killer cells (a type of white

blood cell) from releasing tumor necrosis factor that can damage the placenta and endometrium.

- Reduces the ability of T cells and B cells (white blood cells) to reject the placenta.
- Prevents lymphocytes from wandering into the placenta and causing tissue damage.
- Inhibits prostaglandin production by the uterus, and therefore reduces the risk of uterine contractions during pregnancy.
- Increases the ability of the placenta to produce human chorionic gonadotropin (hCG). This reduces the killing powder of natural killer cells.
- Stimulates the cervix to produce a cervical mucus plug. This is rich in antibodies and prevents microbes from reaching the developing baby and causing infections.

Progesterone is extremely beneficial for all women to use while trying to conceive and during the first trimester of pregnancy. Women with autoimmune disease, allergies or other immune system disorders are advised to use progesterone for the first 16 weeks of pregnancy.

Progesterone can be used as a cream, troches, pessaries or an injection. We recommend progesterone be used in creams, troches or vaginal pessaries. You need a prescription for natural progesterone and daily doses range from 50 to 400 mg. Natural progesterone is referred to as bio-identical because it is molecularly identical to the progesterone made by your own body. This is very different to the synthetic progesterone used in oral contraceptives, hormone replacement therapy or the Mirena IUD.

Thyroid gland disorders and infertility

The thyroid gland is a butterfly shaped gland that sits at the base of your throat, behind your Adam's apple. The thyroid gland is responsible for producing hormones that control growth, metabolism and your energy level. The two main hormones produced by your thyroid gland are T4 and T3. T4 is produced in far higher quantities, but it is largely inactive. T4 is converted into the more potent T3 and this conversion occurs in the thyroid, liver, kidneys, muscle cells and other areas of the body. A large portion of the conversion occurs in the liver, therefore good liver function is essential in order to experience the benefits of thyroid hormones.

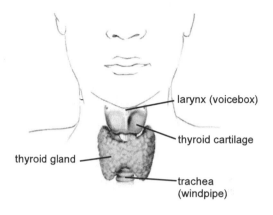

Thyroid problems are incredibly common in women, and undetected and/or inadequately treated thyroid problems are a common cause of infertility in women and men. Thyroid disease also increases the risk of menstrual disorders in women, miscarriage, pregnancy complications, fetal abnormalities and even post-partum depression. Having an under active or over active thyroid gland can result in infertility, however the association is much stronger if you have an under active thyroid.

Subclinical thyroid disease is extremely common and we believe it is responsible for a great deal of infertility in women. Subclinical hypothyroidism is a mildly under active thyroid gland that is usually not diagnosed by most doctors because thyroid hormone levels fall into the supposedly normal range. There is some debate over what the normal range should be, and we will cover this issue in the following section.

Which thyroid disorders can cause infertility?

Any thyroid condition that causes abnormal thyroid hormone levels can result in infertility. Hypothyroidism (under active thyroid) is the most common thyroid abnormality and it has a strong association with infertility. The function of your thyroid gland has an enormous influence on the function of your ovaries. Ovaries contain thyroid hormone receptors and they rely on your thyroid gland to stimulate them to produce adequate hormones required for the function of the menstrual cycle.

Having an over or under active thyroid gland can inhibit ovulation. This disrupts the menstrual cycle and can prevent fertilization. The vast majority of women with a thyroid condition are progesterone deficient. The use of bio-identical progesterone improves the menstrual cycle, increases fertility and improves the function of the thyroid gland. Most thyroid disorders are caused by an autoimmune disease, and the immune dysfunction involved can cause infertility. Most people with a thyroid disease are deficient in iodine, vitamin D, zinc and selenium, and deficiency of any one of these nutrients can cause infertility. As you can see, a thyroid condition can interfere with fertility for a number of reasons.

Symptoms of hypothyroidism

The following symptoms may indicate you have an under active thyroid gland. You may have a few, or all of these symptoms.

- Fatigue
- Weight gain
- Depression
- Increased sensitivity to the cold
- Cold hands and feet
- Constipation
- Dry skin and hair
- Scalp hair loss
- Heavy menstruation and lengthy bleeding (seven plus days)
- Recurrent miscarriages
- Poor concentration and memory
- Muscle weakness, particularly in the arms and legs
- Fluid retention
- Loss of libido

Symptoms of hyperthyroidism

The following symptoms may occur if you have an over active thyroid gland.

- Anxiety
- Insomnia
- Palpitations and rapid heart rate
- Diarrhea or frequent bowel movements
- Tremor
- Intolerance to heat and increased perspiration
- Light menstrual periods, or your period could disappear altogether
- Fatigue
- Shortness of breath
- Eye complaints; particularly gritty or bulging eyes
- Difficulty concentrating

Most of the time people don't have an over active thyroid gland for long. The disease tends to develop quickly and symptoms often become very obvious and unbearable, sending a person off to see their doctor. In the case of an under active thyroid gland though, the symptoms can be milder and may be put down to stress, over work and lack of sleep. Therefore an undiagnosed under active thyroid gland can persist for years, compromising health and fertility.

Autoimmune thyroid disease

Having too much or too little thyroid hormones in your bloodstream can prevent you from falling pregnant, lead to a miscarriage or affect the growth of the fetus. Luckily, with nutritional supplements and medication, we can correct thyroid hormone levels and bring them into the normal range. However, autoimmune thyroid disease is a bigger problem when it comes to infertility. In the vast majority of cases, the thyroid gland becomes over or under active because of autoimmune disease. This means the immune system produces antibodies that either attack and destroy the thyroid (rendering it under active), or antibodies that stimulate it to produce excessive levels of hormones (making the thyroid over active). In the Western world the majority of hypothyroidism is caused by the autoimmune disease Hashimoto's thyroiditis and the majority of hyperthyroidism is caused by Graves' disease. These thyroid diseases are aggravated by nutritional deficiencies, particularly of selenium, iodine, vitamin D and zinc; however, the prime cause of most thyroid dysfunction is autoimmune disease.

Having thyroid antibodies in your bloodstream increases your risk of infertility, miscarriage, premature delivery, intrauterine growth retardation and developmental defects in your baby, particularly cognitive defects and lowered IQ.[19] Women undergoing assisted reproductive technologies (such as IVF) who have thyroid antibodies as well as high-normal TSH levels have a high risk of unsuccessful pregnancy.[20] Having thyroid antibodies in your bloodstream while pregnant increases your risk of postpartum thyroiditis and then hypothyroidism for the rest of your life.

Having thyroid antibodies in your bloodstream is an indicator that all is not well with your immune system. Women with autoimmune thyroid disease are at increased risk of endometriosis and autoimmune premature ovarian failure. These women are also at increased risk of miscarriage, as their immune system may reject the foreign DNA in their fetus.

It is possible to have thyroid antibodies in your bloodstream while having perfectly normal thyroid hormone levels; therefore it is essential that every woman with infertility be tested for thyroid antibodies.

Role of the thyroid gland in pregnancy

The thyroid gland needs to increase its production of thyroid hormones in pregnancy, and this begins by week five. This is so that thyroid hormones are available to your baby before its own thyroid gland is formed. Iodine and selenium are the main minerals required for the production of thyroid hormones. Without adequate levels of these minerals in your diet, your thyroid gland will not be able to step up production of hormones during pregnancy. Women who are taking thyroid hormone medication usually need their dose increased during pregnancy.

Thyroid hormone is essential for the proper development of the placenta, as well as nervous system and brain development of the baby. Deficiency of thyroid hormone during pregnancy can result in mental retardation, decreased intellectual capacity, low IQ, coordination problems, impaired hearing and deafness in the baby. Iodine deficiency is extremely common among women of child bearing age; this is frightening as it places their children at great risk. The amount of iodine excreted in your urine increases during pregnancy, therefore you will need to ingest more iodine to compensate.

Thyroid abnormalities in men

Thyroid disorders are far more common in women, but they do occur in men also. Hyperthyroidism is more common in men than hypothyroidism. Having an over active or under active thyroid gland can reduce the sperm count and cause abnormal sperm motility. These abnormalities improve when thyroid hormone levels are corrected.

Essential blood tests to check for the presence of thyroid disease

TSH, free T4 and free T3 blood test

TSH stands for Thyroid Stimulating Hormone. It is made in the pituitary gland of the brain and it stimulates your thyroid gland to manufacture and release hormones. A low TSH reading indicates your thyroid gland is over active (hyperthyroidism), while a high TSH level indicates your thyroid gland is under active (hypothyroidism). T4 is also known as thyroxine; it is the main hormone made by your thyroid gland. T4 is converted into T3 (also called triiodothyronine), which is the active thyroid hormone.

There is some controversy over the normal range of TSH. The pathology company you visit will likely print a normal range as being 0.3 to 4.5 mIU/L. However, a great deal of research has shown that when TSH reaches 2.5 mIU/L or higher, underlying thyroid disease is already present in the early stages.

In early 2003 new guidelines for thyroid function tests were issued by the American National Academy of Clinical Biochemistry. The normal reference range for TSH was narrowed from 0.5 to 5 mIU/L to 0.3 to 2.5 mIU/L.[21] A review published in the British Medical Journal stated that "thyroid stimulating hormone concentrations above 2 mIU/L are associated with an increased risk of hypothyroidism".[22] Unfortunately most doctors and pathology companies are still not using the updated reference range.

We consider the optimum TSH range to be between 0.3 and 2.5 mIU/L.

Women with a TSH above 2.5 usually take longer to become pregnant, and are at high risk of developing full blown hypothyroidism during their pregnancy. If your TSH is above 2.5, your thyroid may not be able to cope with the increased demand of hormone production during pregnancy. We have found that most of our patients have difficulty getting pregnant unless their TSH is between 0.3 and 2 mIU/L. That seems to be the ideal level. If you are taking thyroid hormone medication, make sure your TSH falls into that range. If not, the dosage of your medication needs to be adjusted.

It is vitally important to have a blood test for free T4 and free T3 as well. This will tell us if your thyroid gland is able to manufacture adequate hormones. The free T3 test will reveal whether your body is converting T4 into its active form T3 adequately. This conversion depends on adequate selenium and also good liver function. See chapter 10 for more detailed information about thyroid blood tests.

Thyroid antibodies blood test

- Thyroid antibodies indicate that an autoimmune disease is present in your body. They are the earliest indicator of a thyroid problem; thyroid antibodies are detectable in the bloodstream long before there is an abnormality in thyroid hormone levels. The presence of thyroid antibodies greatly increases the risk of infertility, miscarriage and poor IVF outcomes, even if thyroid hormone levels are normal. This means it is critical for you to have a blood test for these antibodies, even if your doctor tells you it's irrelevant because you don't have a thyroid disease. Having thyroid antibodies in your bloodstream indicates that your immune system is hyper-stimulated and there is a great deal of inflammation occurring inside your body. This type of immune activity places you at increased risk of developing another autoimmune disease (besides thyroid disease), and at increased risk of rejecting the fetus, leading to a miscarriage.

Urinary iodine test

This test will determine if there is enough iodine in your body. Iodine is a mineral that is the main building block of thyroid hormone. T4 thyroid hormone has four molecules of iodine, while T3 has three. See the following section for dietary sources of iodine.

Overcoming thyroid problems and restoring fertility

• Make sure you obtain enough of the nutrients required for thyroid hormone production; these are iodine, selenium, zinc and tyrosine.

Iodine is predominantly found in the oceans, therefore is in seafood and seaweed. Unfortunately a great deal of seafood available today comes from fish farms. Fish in these farms are not fed their natural diet, therefore their flesh is severely lacking both iodine and omega 3 fats. Apart from seafood, iodized salt, eggs, beans, poultry and potatoes contain small amounts of iodine. Most people get nowhere near enough iodine from their diet; therefore an iodine supplement is essential. We recommend between 160 and 350 micrograms of iodine per day.

Iodine deficiency can make your thyroid under active and leave you feeling tired and sluggish. Losing weight will be more difficult if you are iodine deficient. Long term severe iodine deficiency can cause the thyroid gland to swell and form a goiter.

Selenium is a mineral that is very deficient in the soils of many parts of the world; therefore it is very difficult to obtain enough of this vital mineral through your diet. Selenium is required for the production, activation and metabolism of thyroid hormone. A healthy thyroid gland contains more selenium per gram than any other tissue in the body. Selenium is required by the enzyme that converts T4 thyroid hormone into its active form T3. If you are selenium deficient you will not be able to manufacture sufficient T3 and you may experience the symptoms of an under active thyroid. Selenium deficiency can cause your body to manufacture excessively high levels of the inactive form of T3 called reverse T3.

Selenium deficiency greatly increases the risk of autoimmune thyroid disease, such as Hashimoto's thyroiditis, Graves' disease and postpartum thyroiditis. In fact selenium deficiency increases the risk of all types of autoimmune disease, and several autoimmune diseases have been shown to increase the risk of infertility and miscarriage. This subject is covered in more detail in chapter 5. Selenium has an anti-inflammatory effect and can inhibit the production of antibodies that attack your own organs and tissues. If a test has shown you have thyroid antibodies in your bloodstream, it is vital you take a selenium supplement. The required daily dose of selenium needed to stop auto-antibody production is 200 micrograms per day. It is virtually impossible to obtain this level of selenium through food, because very few foods are a good source of this mineral. Brazil nuts, garlic and seafood contain some selenium.

Vitamin D is a hormone-like substance that is produced in the skin during exposure to sunlight. You are probably aware that vitamin D is required for strong bones and the prevention of osteoporosis, but this vitamin has countless other vital functions in your body. Recent research has shown that vitamin D is essential for a strong and healthy immune system. According to the Vitamin D Council in California, USA, vitamin D deficiency increases the risk of at least 17 different types of cancer.

Vitamin D deficiency also increases the risk of autoimmune disease, including autoimmune thyroid disease. Deficiency of this vitamin is a major trigger for the development of Hashimoto's thyroiditis, Graves' disease and postpartum thyroiditis. Vitamin D has a strong anti-inflammatory effect and if you have autoimmune thyroid disease, it is essential that you obtain sufficient quantities of this vitamin.

Surprisingly vitamin D deficiency is very common in sunny Australia. A study conducted in 2001 detected mild or moderate vitamin D deficiency in more than one in three women during summer, and one in two in winter.[23]

You will need to have a blood test for vitamin D to determine how much you should be taking in supplement form. There is more information about vitamin D on page 89.

Tyrosine is an amino acid (building block of protein) that is essential for the formation of thyroid hormones. Tyrosine is found in protein rich foods such as red meat, poultry and eggs, as well as bananas and avocados. Your body can also manufacture tyrosine out of another amino acid called phenylalanine. For these reasons, most people obtain adequate tyrosine in their diet for thyroid hormone production. Vegetarians, people with poor digestion and people taking stomach acid suppressing medication are at increased risk of tyrosine deficiency. Stress depletes your body of tyrosine.

Zinc is required for the formation of thyroid hormone and the conversion of T4 hormone into its active form T3. Zinc deficiency is extremely common and this can make you more prone to infections, and cause white spots to appear on your finger nails.

The most important nutrients required for the thyroid gland are found in **Thyroid Health capsules**.

- Avoid consuming very large quantities of raw vegetables in the brassica (cruciferous) family; these include cabbage, broccoli, cauliflower and Brussels sprouts. These vegetables contain goitrogens, which are substances that impair the thyroid gland from absorbing and utilizing iodine. Cooking inactivates the majority of goitrogens.
- Keep your intake of soy to a minimum. Soy can also inhibit the thyroid gland from using iodine. It tends to make iodine deficiency worse, which is a problem because so many people are already iodine deficient.
- If you are taking thyroid hormone, make sure your TSH falls between 0.3 and 2 mIU/L. Make sure you have a blood test for free T3 to ensure that your body is utilizing the medication correctly. If you do not feel well on thyroxine (brand name Synthroid), there are alternatives. You may need to take T3 as well as thyroxine and the brand name for this is Cytomel. You may want to try porcine thyroid extract or bio-identical thyroid hormones, which are available from compounding pharmacies. See our book *Your Thyroid Problems Solved* for much more detailed information about the treatment of thyroid disease.

- If a blood test has shown you have thyroid antibodies, you need to follow our treatment plan for autoimmune disease. This involves following a gluten and dairy free diet, eliminating other food allergens and taking some anti-inflammatory supplements. See our recommendations for reducing auto-antibodies and calming inflammation in chapter 5 .
- Drink filtered tap water, as chlorine and fluoride in tap water can compete for absorption with iodine. This means your thyroid gland will have less iodine available for thyroid hormone production. Avoid fluoride containing toothpaste.
- Minimize your exposure to radiation, pesticides and chemicals, as many have been found to interfere with thyroid hormone production and increase the risk of autoimmune thyroid disease. See chapter 9 for information on minimizing your exposure to chemicals.
- Fish oil and probiotics (beneficial bowel bacteria) are both excellent natural anti-inflammatories that calm down an overstimulated immune system. This is important if you have autoimmune thyroid disease.

Important Points to Remember

Your TSH may be in the so called normal range, but it needs to be in the optimal range to optimize your fertility; that is 0.3 to 2 mIU/L.

Check to see if you have thyroid antibodies in your bloodstream. If you do, you have an autoimmune disease and must follow our treatment plan for autoimmune disease in chapter 5

Ensure you receive optimal levels of the nutrients required for a healthy thyroid gland; these are iodine, selenium, vitamin D and zinc.

If you have any questions about our recommendations, please phone Dr Cabot's Health Advisory Line in Australia on 02 4655 8855 or the United States of America on 623 334 3232 or email contact@weightcontroldoctor.com. If you have a thyroid problem, you will find far more detailed information on how to overcome it in our book *Your Thyroid Problems Solved.*

Case study: thyroid disease and infertility

Denise was a slim and anxious 26 year old lady who came to see me because she could not conceive after 12 months of trying. She was very health conscious, took several nutritional supplements and exercised regularly. Unfortunately Denise was an extremely anxious person and anxiety ran in her family.

Denise also had Graves' disease (over active thyroid). This was a very recent diagnosis and the only medication her doctor put her on was a beta blocker in order to slow her heart rate. She had only mild symptoms of hyperthyroidism and Denise wanted to resolve it naturally before trying medication. Denise's doctor already had her on progesterone cream, which she used for the second half of her menstrual cycle and which helped her enormously.

Firstly I placed Denise on a gluten and dairy free diet. This was essential because Graves' disease is an autoimmune disease. Denise's immune system was stimulating her thyroid gland to produce abnormally high levels of hormones. I also put Denise on a magnesium powder; this had a wonderfully relaxing effect on her and helped her to sleep better. Denise was vitamin D deficient; therefore she was given a supplement. I also gave her selenium, fish oil and B vitamins.

When I saw Denise again four weeks later, she appeared much calmer and said that she felt much less overwhelmed with life in general. Her energy levels were much better and she no longer experienced abdominal bloating or gas. Eight weeks later a blood test revealed that Denise's thyroid hormones had returned back into the normal range, therefore she was technically no longer suffering with hyperthyroidism. Her thyroid antibodies also returned to normal. I took Denise off the beta blocker as she no longer required it.

I ordered a urine test for Denise which revealed iodine deficiency. The multivitamin she had always taken only contained 31 mcg of iodine; therefore I gave her an additional 160 mcg. Denise was still struggling with anxiety; therefore she took up yoga classes and found that helped immensely. However, a month after that she found a new job and that had a profound effect on her peace of mind. Much of the stress in her life was surrounding her job; resigning lifted a huge load off her shoulders.

Five months after I first saw Denise, her health was excellent and there were no known factors that were impairing her fertility. However, Denise wanted to delay trying to conceive for another few months because she worried that a pregnancy may cause her thyroid condition to return. Therefore it was five months later that I received a call from Denise telling me she is pregnant. I saw her several times throughout her pregnancy, and adjusted her progesterone cream and supplements as necessary. Denise had a healthy baby boy.

4. Structural factors in women responsible for infertility

Blocked fallopian tubes account for approximately 20 percent of cases of female infertility. This condition is often referred to as tubal factor infertility. The fallopian tubes (also known as the oviduct) are two tubes, approximately ten centimeters long that carry eggs between the ovaries and uterus. The tubes are roughly the thickness of spaghetti. The inner lining of the tubes contains tiny hair-like structures called cilia; they help the egg move along the tube towards the uterus. The tubes also secrete mucus, which helps the egg to easily slide along the tube. Because these tubes are extremely narrow, even a minor blockage can create a big problem.

How do blocked fallopian tubes cause infertility?

Blocked fallopian tubes prevent the sperm and egg from being able to meet. At ovulation one egg is released from an ovary and travels down the fallopian tube towards the uterus. Sperm travel from the cervix, into the uterus and up the fallopian tubes in search of an egg. A blockage will prevent them from being able to meet. Sometimes if there is only a partial blockage, the sperm and egg do meet, but they can't travel to the uterus and implant in the uterine wall. This can result in an ectopic pregnancy (a pregnancy where the fertilized egg implants somewhere else, not the uterus). An ectopic pregnancy is a medical emergency and requires medication or surgical intervention. Unfortunately it can lead to complete destruction of a fallopian tube. For this reason we recommend that you have a pelvic ultrasound as soon as a blood test confirms you are pregnant. This is essential to make sure that the embryo is growing in the correct location (the uterus). Women with a history of infertility are at higher risk of ectopic pregnancy.

It is interesting to note that blocked fallopian tubes was the main reason why IVF was initially developed and used. Basically plumbing problems were the original reason couples sought

IVF. These days couples undergo IVF for a myriad of reasons, the majority of which can be solved with nutritional medicine.

What causes blocked fallopian tubes?

The problem is that blocked fallopian tubes usually cause no symptoms or problems, until a women tries to fall pregnant. If only one tube is blocked, a successful pregnancy can usually be achieved, but it often takes longer to fall pregnant. The fallopian tubes can become severely blocked by factors such as scar tissue, or they can become temporarily clogged with mucus. Tubes that are blocked with mucus can usually be cleared with the use of diet changes and nutritional medicine. A number of factors can cause blocked fallopian tubes, including:

• Scarring from endometriosis
• Scarring as a result of pelvic inflammatory disease (PID), caused by infection or immune mediated inflammation
• Complications from IUD use, such as removal due to pain, bleeding or infection
• Previous sexually transmitted infection, particularly chlamydia or gonorrhoea.
• Previous uterine infection caused by miscarriage or pregnancy termination
• Abdominal surgery in the past
• Previous ectopic pregnancy
• Ruptured appendix in the past
• Autoimmune disease
• Food allergy or intolerance. Eating foods that don't agree with you can lead to excess mucus production throughout your body.
• Dehydration. Not drinking enough water can make the mucus in your fallopian tubes more thick and sticky.
• Pharmaceutical drugs. Antihistamines, dry cough liquids and some cold and flu medicine can make the mucus thicker.

Blocked tubes as a result of mucus can usually be corrected with a change of diet. See chapter 8 for our diet recommendations. Hydrosalpinx is a specific kind of blockage where the tube dilates and fills with fluid. In some cases, hydrosalpinx can cause lower abdominal pain and a vaginal discharge.

The most common test to check whether the fallopian tubes are blocked or not is called a hysterosalpingogram (HSG). This test involves inserting a dye into the cervix, which travels up through the fallopian tubes. Once the dye has been inserted, an X ray is taken of the pelvis. We do not recommend this test, as it exposes the ovaries to radiation. Another test called a hysterosalpingo contrast sonogram is available, and is preferable because it uses an ultrasound. While this test is being performed, the fallopian tubes can be rinsed with a saline solution. This can help to clear minor blockages.

How to overcome blocked fallopian tubes

In severe cases of blockage, laparoscopic surgery is done in an attempt to open blocked tubes and remove scar tissue. Occasionally stents are used to try and open the tubes. These methods are usually not terribly successful, therefore the focus needs to be on preventing the tubes from becoming blocked in the first place. This is not always possible of course, but some conditions (particularly endometriosis and sexually transmitted infections) are notorious for creating blocked tubes if left untreated. Therefore these conditions must be diagnosed and treated as soon as possible, to prevent them causing irreparable harm to the reproductive tract.

Minor blockages can be overcome with the following strategies:

- If you have the symptoms of endometriosis, get a diagnosis and follow our recommended treatment. The longer endometriosis is allowed to persist, the more harm it does to the reproductive tract.
- Be tested for sexually transmitted infections if you have sex with a new partner. Many STIs cause no symptoms, but they can cause structural damage to the reproductive system if left untreated.
- To minimize the chances of thick mucus blocking the fallopian tubes, avoid consuming dairy products and any other food you may be sensitive or intolerant to. Common culprits include wheat, gluten, soy, nuts and yeast. A high sugar and refined carbohydrate intake also creates excess mucus production.

- Include spices in your diet such as cinnamon, chilli, garlic and ginger, as they improve circulation to the pelvic organs.
- Drink plenty of purified water, herbal tea or green tea.

Adhesions and scarring

Adhesions are a type of scar tissue that usually forms as a result of injury, infection or surgery. Adhesions in the reproductive organs can impair ovarian function, block fallopian tubes, or prevent implantation of an embryo in the uterus. The most common causes of adhesions are endometriosis, appendicitis and pelvic inflammatory disease. The latter is usually caused by a sexually transmitted infection that was not treated promptly. The longer any of these diseases are left to progress, the worse the adhesions can become.

Women with adhesions on or around their fallopian tubes are at greater risk of infertility and ectopic pregnancy. Adhesions that form within the uterus can cause infertility or repeated miscarriage. These kinds of adhesions are commonly referred to as Asherman's syndrome or uterine synechiae. Adhesions can form after a D & C (dilation and curettage). This is a common procedure, performed on women with heavy, continual menstrual bleeding, or used to clear the uterus after childbirth, miscarriage or pregnancy termination. D & C is a very commonly performed procedure and it is estimated that five percent of procedures lead to adhesions.

How to reduce the risk of adhesions

Some people naturally produce a lot more scar tissue than others, and this is determined by their genes. The following points can help to reduce excess scar tissue:

- Make sure you receive prompt treatment of diseases that can cause adhesions. If you experience very painful menstrual cramps, or have abdominal or pelvic discomfort at other times of the month, go to your doctor early for a diagnosis.
- Avoid contracting a sexually transmitted infection.
- Zinc, MSM and vitamin E help to soften scar tissue. These are best taken in supplement form if you already have adhesions, as your diet will not provide enough of these nutrients.

Ectopic pregnancy

An ectopic pregnancy is a pregnancy that develops in a location other than the uterus. Most commonly it occurs in the fallopian tubes, but it may also occur in the cervix, in an ovary or in the abdominal cavity. Conception occurs when the sperm penetrates the egg in a fallopian tube. Normally the fertilized egg then travels down the fallopian tube and implants in the uterine wall.

Symptoms of ectopic pregnancy

In the initial stages, an ectopic pregnancy mimics the symptoms of a normal pregnancy. Most women experience a little morning sickness and breast tenderness. However, the following symptoms soon develop:

- Lower abdominal pain
- Lower back pain
- Cramps on one side of the abdomen
- Vaginal bleeding or spotting
- If a fallopian tube ruptures there is severe pain in the lower abdomen. This is a medical emergency and requires immediate surgery.

Risk factors for ectopic pregnancy

Women with infertility are at increased risk of having an ectopic pregnancy. It generally occurs when there is a blockage in a fallopian tube, or the tiny hair-like structures (cilia) in the tubes cannot move the fertilized egg along properly. The following factors increase the risk of ectopic pregnancy:

- Previous infection of the pelvic organs and fallopian tubes
- Endometriosis
- Progesterone deficiency
- Reversal of a tubal ligation
- Surgery to remove the appendix
- Cigarette smoking. Smoking quadruples the risk of ectopic pregnancy. This is because it increases levels of a protein called PROKR1 in the fallopian tubes. This substance inhibits movement of the egg along the fallopian tube.

Ectopic pregnancies that are detected at an advanced stage require surgery to remove the embryo and attempt to repair the fallopian tube. In non-emergency cases, medication is usually given to induce a miscarriage. Women who have had one ectopic pregnancy are at risk of having another.

An ectopic pregnancy can do a great deal of harm to your fertility, mainly through destruction of a fallopian tube. Therefore, as soon as a blood test confirms you are pregnant, we strongly recommend you have an ultrasound to confirm that the embryo is developing in your uterus, where it should be.

5. Immune system disorders that lead to infertility

A great number of immune system disorders have the potential to cause infertility, miscarriage and pregnancy complications. Some of these are well known, such as lupus and premature ovarian failure, whereas in others the link is not so obvious. We believe that subtle immune system disorders are responsible for a large number of so called unexplained infertility. Once the immune system is restored to a healthy state, many couples are able to achieve conception and a healthy pregnancy.

In this chapter we will look at the various immune system disorders one by one, outlining the symptoms and necessary diagnostic tests. However, regardless which antibodies are being produced, the treatment of immune system disorders that lead to infertility is the same. All immune system disorders produce excess inflammation in the body, and this must be addressed.

What is autoimmune disease?

The term autoimmune disease refers to more than 80 different diseases. Some are severe and life threatening, while others are mild. Autoimmune disease can affect nearly every organ and tissue in the body. In each autoimmune disease, the body's immune system becomes misdirected and starts attacking and destroying parts of the body. Women are far more susceptible to getting an autoimmune disease than men, and in fact approximately 75 percent of autoimmune disease occurs in women. Some examples of autoimmune diseases are lupus, multiple sclerosis, type 1 diabetes, vitiligo, rheumatoid arthritis, Crohn's disease and ulcerative colitis, pernicious anemia and psoriasis.

People with an autoimmune disease have a great deal of inflammation occurring inside their bodies. The chemicals released by immune cells cause wear and tear to organs and tissues, and some autoimmune diseases can increase the risk of blood clots. People with one autoimmune disease are at high risk of developing another one. It is interesting to note that women with autoimmune disease are at greater risk of having an autistic child.

All autoimmune disease increases the risk of infertility and miscarriage, however on the following pages we will describe which diseases are most strongly associated with these conditions.

Premature ovarian failure

Premature ovarian failure means the ovaries are no longer able to produce eggs or sufficient hormones before the age of 40. It is essentially a premature menopause and occurs in between one and four percent of women. Most women are born with enough eggs in their ovaries to last them all the way up to menopause, which occurs at an average age of 54. While you were growing inside your mother's uterus, you had a maximum of seven millions eggs. From then onwards, the number of eggs you have starts to drop, and the eggs cannot be replaced. By the time you are born, the number of eggs inside your ovaries has dropped to approximately two million. By the time you have your first period, the number of eggs you have has diminished to approximately 400 thousand.[24]

The normal wear and tear of life causes the eggs inside your ovaries to deteriorate, but cigarette smoking and an unhealthy lifestyle speed up the destruction of eggs. In fact smoking cigarettes ages a woman's ovaries by up to ten years. Often women in their mid 30s decide they'd like to have a baby, therefore quit smoking. Unfortunately the damage has often already been done.

In women with premature ovarian failure, something has happened to cause the eggs to be destroyed at far too young an age. Premature ovarian failure is also called premature menopause, premature ovarian insufficiency and hypergonadotropic amenorrhea.

Symptoms of premature ovarian failure (POF)

Women with POF stop having menstrual periods, or periods become irregular or infrequent. The following symptoms may also be present:

- Hot flushes
- Night sweats
- Poor sleep
- Mood swings
- Vaginal dryness
- Bladder weakness

Premature ovarian failure basically causes menopause symptoms. In some women symptoms can be severe, whereas other women experience minimal symptoms or no symptoms at all.

What causes premature ovarian failure?

In most cases, premature ovarian failure is an autoimmune disease. The immune system attacks the ovaries, leaving them unable to produce adequate hormones or eggs. People with one autoimmune disease are prone to developing others, and there is a strong association between POF and the following autoimmune diseases:

Addison's disease (adrenal insufficiency)

Autoimmune thyroid disease

Rheumatoid arthritis

Hypoparathyroidism

Idiopathic thrombocytopaenia (ITP)

Type 1 diabetes

Pernicious anemia

Vitiligo

Systemic lupus erythematosus (SLE)

Polyglandular failure I and II

Women with any of those diseases are at increased risk of having a premature, early menopause before age 40.

Other potential causes of premature ovarian failure include:

- Genetic diseases (eg. Turner syndrome)
- Metabolic diseases (eg. galactosemia, hemochromatosis, thalassemia)

- Chemotherapy and radiotherapy
- Viral infections
- Heavy cigarette smoking and/or recreational drug use
- Severe nutritional deficiencies, underweight and anorexia nervosa
- Ovarian drilling for polycystic ovarian syndrome

Diagnosis of premature ovarian failure

A blood test for follicle stimulating hormone (FSH) is the initial test used to determine ovarian function. In pre-menopausal women FSH is below 15 mIU/L. Women with premature ovarian failure typically have an FSH level above 40 mIU/L. FSH is manufactured in the brain, and a high reading indicates that the ovaries are not responding to the brain's request to manufacture hormones. FSH must be tested on at least two occasions, six weeks apart to confirm the diagnosis. Other tests are then ordered, including estrogen and progesterone blood tests, an ultrasound of the ovaries and blood tests for genetic abnormalities. If the premature ovarian failure is caused by autoimmune disease, anti-ovarian antibodies will be present in the bloodstream.

Consequences of premature ovarian failure

Experiencing an early menopause places women at increased risk of osteoporosis, heart attacks and strokes. Luckily these conditions can be managed with the use of natural hormones, diet and lifestyle improvements and nutritional supplements. Infertility is the most devastating consequence of POF. Typically the condition strikes in the mid 30s, when many women are just ready to start a family. Approximately six to eight percent of women with POF are able to conceive naturally. This figure is probably much higher if the condition is detected early and the health of the immune system is restored. Many women with premature ovarian failure need to use a donor egg if they want to be pregnant.

Celiac disease

Research has found that between four and eight percent of women with unexplained infertility have undiagnosed celiac disease.[25] Celiac disease is also known as gluten intolerance. It is an autoimmune disease triggered by the ingestion of gluten.

Gluten is found in wheat, rye, oats, barley, spelt, kamut and many processed foods under names like starch, maltodextrin or thickeners.

When people with celiac disease eat gluten, the immune cells in their digestive tract respond as though the person ingested a harmful virus or bacteria. The immune system mounts an attack on the gluten and this causes inflammation and tissue damage in the digestive tract. This inflammation compromises the integrity of the digestive lining; it makes it more permeable, or leaky. This situation promotes widespread systemic inflammation, increased allergies and greatly increases the risk of other autoimmune diseases. People with celiac disease have many vitamin, mineral and essential fatty acid deficiencies because their digestion is so disrupted that they can't digest food thoroughly. The nutrient deficiencies further contribute to infertility.

Removing all traces of gluten from the diet, restoring the intestinal lining and assisting the immune system will completely restore the health of a person with celiac disease. The problem is the majority of people with celiac disease are not aware they have it. Traditionally celiac disease was diagnosed with a blood test and intestinal biopsy (to check for intestinal damage). However, we now know that celiac disease is just one manifestation of gluten intolerance. Not every gluten intolerant person has intestinal damage. Gluten can cause harm to other parts of the body. An elimination diet, genetic tests, blood tests and the presence of autoimmune disease are all potentially useful diagnostic indicators of gluten intolerance. It is best to consult a naturopath or your doctor for help with a diagnosis.

Undiagnosed celiac disease is strongly associated with infertility and adverse pregnancy outcomes. Celiacs typically experience late menarche (first menstrual period), premature menopause, amenorrhea (loss of menstrual periods), recurrent miscarriages,[26] low birth weight babies, premature babies[27] and problems with breast feeding.[28] Sticking to a gluten free diet greater reduces the risk of these complications. Men with celiac disease are also at increased risk of infertility.

Autoimmune diseases associated with infertility

Autoimmune thyroid disease

The presence of thyroid antibodies in your bloodstream is associated with infertility. Having antibodies in your bloodstream against any organ or tissue is a marker of systemic inflammation and an over-stimulated immune system that can sabotage successful pregnancy. Thyroid disease is covered in more detail in chapter 3.

Anti-phospholipid syndrome

Anti-phospholipid syndrome is an autoimmune disease characterized by recurring blood clots (thromboses). It is sometimes referred to as Hughes syndrome. The blood clots can occur in any blood vessel of the body. The symptoms and severity of this disease are largely determined by where the blood clots occur. Sometimes anti-phospholipid syndrome occurs on its own, and sometimes it occurs with another autoimmune disease, particularly systemic lupus erythematosis. The increased tendency to form blood clots is called thrombophilia. It can be caused by autoimmune disease or inherited blood clotting disorders.

Phospholipids are molecules that make up cell membranes, and antibodies against these molecules can be detected in the bloodstream of sufferers. Women with anti-phospholipid syndrome are prone to developing blood clots in arteries of the uterus. Clots here interrupt the blood supply to the embryo and can result in miscarriage. The miscarriage may occur at the earliest stages of pregnancy, so that the woman wasn't even aware she was pregnant.

Sometimes the miscarriage occurs at a later stage of pregnancy. Because the placenta differs from other tissues in your body, it is at particularly high risk of damage from anti-phospholipid antibodies. Women with anti-phospholipid syndrome are also significantly more likely to develop pre-eclampsia and eclampsia during pregnancy, restricted fetal growth and pre-term delivery. Pre-eclampsia is pregnancy-induced high blood pressure and it is covered in chapter 7. The conventional treatment of anti-phospholipid syndrome is to give pregnant women a low dose of aspirin or the blood thinning drug heparin. Unfortunately these therapies are not always effective.

Systemic lupus erythematosis (SLE)

Lupus is an autoimmune disease that is far more common in women than men, and it is usually diagnosed during the childbearing years. The immune system produces antibodies that attack and destroy connective tissue. This causes a great deal of inflammation in the body and symptoms vary depending on which body parts are affected. Commonly lupus affects the joints, skin and kidneys. Lupus can be mild or life threatening. People with lupus have several antibodies in their bloodstream, including antinuclear antibodies, smooth muscle antibodies and cardiolipin antibodies. Women with lupus anticoagulant antibodies are most prone to infertility and pregnancy complications. Blood tests for these antibodies can be organized by an immunologist or your GP. Having these antibodies in your bloodstream indicates that you are at higher risk of blood clots in arteries of the placenta, inflammation of the placenta, and subsequent infertility or miscarriage. High levels of inflammation may be present around the embryo at the time of implantation, or in the placenta after implantation.

In the past, women with autoimmune disease were generally advised not to become pregnant. These days a lot more is known about autoimmune disease and there are effective ways to manage the disease in most instances. If you have lupus and are wishing to fall pregnant, it is vital that you are in remission at the time. This will reduce the risk of harm to you and your baby. Interestingly, women with lupus who do become pregnant are at risk of thyroiditis (inflamed thyroid gland) during pregnancy. Therefore it is vital to have regular thyroid hormone blood tests during pregnancy, as well as blood tests for thyroid antibodies. One study showed that one out of every three pregnant women with lupus has thyroid disease before, during or after pregnancy.[29]

Some medication used in the treatment of lupus can suppress fertility, and high doses of steroids can stop menstrual periods. Women with lupus are more prone to developing pre-eclampsia and eclampsia in pregnancy and approximately 25 percent of pregnancies end in miscarriage or stillbirth. Approximately 25 percent of births are premature. A small percentage of babies born to mothers with lupus develop neonatal lupus. This is a temporary condition and usually disappears by the time the infant is three to six months old. Approximately half of babies born with neonatal lupus are born with a heart condition. This is permanent and can be treated with a pacemaker. It is vital that all women with autoimmune disease follow our inflammation reducing recommendations later in this chapter.

Allergies and your immune system

Allergy, intolerance or sensitivity to foods, chemicals and other substances is on the rise. Sometimes allergies cause obvious symptoms, such as eczema, hay fever or a digestive upset shortly after coming into contact with a substance; but at other times the reaction is far more subtle and harder to detect. If you are sensitive to a food, airborne substance (such as pollen, grass or dust mites) or chemical, it means you have an over reactive immune system. Your immune system is responding to substances that should be harmless. You would have inherited the allergic tendency from one or both of your parents, but environmental factors are required in order to trigger off the allergic reaction.

Allergies can cause strange and unusual symptoms that you probably would not recognize as being caused by allergies. The following list describes possible allergy symptoms:

Respiratory system: asthma, hay fever, runny nose (rhinitis), post-nasal drip (mucus running down the back of the throat), blocked nose, particularly at night, chronic cough, sore throat or itchy throat.

Ears and eyes: blocked ears, repeated ear infections, red ears, particularly after a meal, runny eyes, conjunctivitis, sensitivity to light, gritty or itchy eyes, eczema on or around the eyes.

Digestive system: diarrhea, constipation, irritable bowel syndrome, abdominal bloating, flatulence, burping, abdominal cramps, heartburn, reflux, nausea, indigestion.

Urinary system: frequent night time urination, urinary incontinence, weak bladder, interstitial cystitis.

Emotional: anxiety, depression, fatigue, particularly after meals, poor concentration, restlessness, insomnia or frequent night time waking, hyperactivity.

Muscular and skeletal: joint pain, muscle aches, muscle cramps, weak muscles.

Skin: eczema, dermatitis, hives, flushed cheeks, itchy skin, dandruff, dark rings under the eyes.

Miscellaneous: Low grade fever, night time perspiration, headaches (including migraines), rapid pulse, heart palpitations, bad breath, excessive vaginal discharge, hypoglycemia.

This is quite a long list, and many of these symptoms can be caused by other conditions. However, if you suffer with at least four of these symptoms, there is a high probability that you have an allergy or sensitivity to foods and/or chemicals. Being an allergy sufferer means you have high levels of inflammation inside your body. Each time your immune system comes in contact with a food or other substance you are sensitive to, your immune cells release a flood of inflammatory chemicals. These chemicals cause wear and tear inside your body and can compromise the health of your organs and tissues. This is why allergies can produce such varied symptoms in nearly any part of the body.

Allergy sufferers are at increased risk of infertility, as the excess inflammation in the body can cause implantation problems and miscarriage. Immune system disorders are a common cause of unexplained infertility. It is important to fix your immune system and address your allergies, in order to prevent passing on the allergic tendency to your children. Unless your immune system function is improved, allergies increase your risk of developing autoimmune disease.

Why are allergies so common?

Allergies are an over reaction by the immune system to substances that are normally harmless. Allergy, intolerance and sensitivity to foods, chemicals, drugs and other substances are definitely on the rise. One possible explanation is the Hygiene Hypothesis. This was first proposed in 1989 and states that the increasing prevalence of allergies is due to a child's reduced exposure to germs during infancy and childhood. This is largely due to declining family size, reduced exposure to animals in childhood, and higher standards of cleanliness in homes. In our modern world, pathogenic bacteria have been replaced with pollutants and chemicals. Therefore, today's children experience far fewer infections, yet are plagued with eczema, asthma, hay fever and food intolerance.

Research has shown that children who grow up on farms are far less likely to develop allergies. The presence of intestinal worms also guards against allergies, as children in developing nations (where intestinal worms are endemic) rarely develop allergies. It is also interesting to note that infants born via caesarian section are at increased risk of celiac disease, asthma and allergies. This is probably because these children miss out on exposure to beneficial bacteria in the birth canal. This is concerning, given the fact that one in three babies born in Queensland, Australia is delivered via caesarean section.[30]

You are more likely to have allergies if your mother ate things she was allergic to while you were inside her womb. Allergies can also occur if solids are introduced into an infant's diet too soon (earlier than six months), particularly dairy products and gluten. Solids introduced into an immature digestive tract cannot be broken down properly, consequently whole food molecules get absorbed into the bloodstream. Immune cells in the bloodstream recognize these foreign molecules and this triggers an allergic reaction. Eczema and asthma are common in infancy and childhood and many children supposedly outgrow these allergic diseases. In fact they don't outgrow them at all, they just change form. Eczema and asthma commonly develop into hay fever, allergic rhinitis (runny nose) or sinusitis. Sometimes allergies die down for years and re-emerge following a stressful life episode or infection. Irritable bowel syndrome is common in people who had childhood allergies.

How to reduce the risk of allergies in your children

The tendency to have allergies is inherited, therefore if you or your partner have allergies, your children are at higher risk of having them also. However, allergies are so common nowadays that we frequently come across children with multiple allergies, with parents who have none. The most common symptoms of allergies in children are skin rashes, runny nose, blocked nose, sleeping with the mouth open, snoring, constipation or diarrhea, bloated abdomen, poor sleep and a restless infant that is difficult to settle. Food allergies in an infant can make your life difficult and inconvenient, but they can also be life threatening for your child. Fortunately, a great deal of research has shown that certain nutrients can help to protect your child's immune system from developing allergies. Before and during your pregnancy, the food you eat and the nutrients you consume will have a profound effect on your child's immune system.

• **Avoid consuming foods you are allergic or intolerant to**

Before and during pregnancy, you need to avoid eating foods that you know or suspect make you feel unwell. Inflammatory chemicals produced in your body as a result of food intolerance can pass through the placenta and affect your developing baby's immune system. Dairy products and gluten are the most common cause of overt and subtle immune reactions; therefore we recommend you avoid those foods before and during pregnancy. In some people nuts, soy, eggs, yeast or other foods can be problematic. It is best to see a naturopath to help you identify your potentially problematic foods.

• **Take fish oil**

Due to modern agricultural methods, it is virtually impossible to get enough omega 3 fats in your diet. The fatty acids in fish are strongly anti-inflammatory and help to dampen down an overactive immune system. A team of German researchers studied the incidence of eczema in 2641 children at two years of age. The scientists found that a high intake of omega 3 fats during the last four weeks of pregnancy was associated with a much lower incidence of eczema during the first two years of life.[31]

In another study, 145 pregnant women with a family history of allergies were given 1.6 g of EPA and 1.1 g of DHA or a placebo beginning at the 25th week of pregnancy until three to four months of breast-feeding. The prevalence of food allergies and IgE mediated eczema was significantly lower in the infants whose mother received fish oil.[32]

- **Vitamin D**

This is the most important vitamin for reducing the risk of allergies and autoimmune disease. The Finnish Type 1 Diabetes Prediction and Prevention Nutrition Study was conducted on 931 children who were monitored for five years. Researchers discovered that maternal intake of vitamin D during pregnancy was strongly protective against the development of food allergies in offspring.[33] An American study has shown that early correction of vitamin D deficiency can promote healthy bowel bacteria in infants, a healthier digestive lining and less susceptibility to allergies.[34]

- **Probiotics**

Probiotics (good bowel bacteria) are well known for their ability to prevent and even treat allergies in children and adults. A recent review of five studies, involving 1477 babies found significant benefits of probiotic supplements, especially those containing L. rhamnosus. The infants in these studies were known to be at particularly high risk of allergies. Use of probiotic supplements in pregnant women significantly reduces the risk of eczema and allergies in offspring and the benefits last up to four years.[35]

How inflammation can cause infertility

Inflammation is generally a consequence of how the body protects itself from harmful microorganisms and allergens (allergy inducing substances). It is a reaction by your immune system to injury, infection or irritation. The main symptoms of inflammation are redness, heat, swelling and pain. Loss of mobility is also sometimes present. Think of a sprained ankle or a gout attack in a toe; those conditions both cause obvious inflammation. The inflammation is intense and short lived. The inflammatory chemicals that are produced by immune cells have important functions and enable your body to recover from whatever caused the tissue damage.

Inflammation can also occur in a far more subtle way in your body, whereby you are unaware of its presence. We know that chronic low grade inflammation is extremely common and it is behind a range of chronic health problems. Inflammation that is allowed to persist causes wear and tear and free radical damage to your cells, organs and tissues. Chronic inflammation is thought to be behind the development of heart disease and strokes (because of damage done to artery walls), cancer, osteoporosis, arthritis and nearly every (if not every) chronic disease. Chronic inflammation increases the risk of autoimmune disease, and people with autoimmune disease have extremely high levels of inflammatory chemicals in their bodies. The conventional treatment of inflammation involves the use of steroids and non-steroidal anti-inflammatory drugs (NSAIDs). Examples of NSAIDs are aspirin, ibuprofen and naproxen; all extremely commonly prescribed drugs. Examples of steroids are cortisone tablets, cortisone cream and some asthma preventative inhalers.

One reason why inflammation is so wide spread is because the Western diet is so pro-inflammatory. Sugar, flour, dairy products, alcohol and vegetable oil are all highly inflammatory foods. Combine that with sedentary lifestyles, air pollution and chronic stress and you have a body brimming with harmful inflammatory chemicals.

People with high levels of inflammation in their bodies tend to over react to normally harmless substances. Therefore they are prone to reacting to foods, pollens, grass and animal hair. This can pose a challenge when trying to fall pregnant. When a woman is pregnant, her immune system must learn to be tolerant of a "foreign body" growing inside her. If you think about it, half of the fetus growing inside a pregnant woman is technically "non-self", meaning it contains DNA from the father. Our bodies are normally designed to destroy foreign tissue (which is what makes organ donation so difficult). In a healthy woman, her immune system is somewhat suppressed during pregnancy in order to prevent immune cells from destroying the "foreign body" inside her uterus. This state is described as immune tolerance. Women with an over stimulated immune system may lose this ability. Their fetus is at increased risk of being destroyed by the immune system.

What do all autoimmune diseases and allergies have in common? Leaky gut syndrome

You have probably heard of leaky gut syndrome. It basically means that the lining of the small intestine has become more permeable than it should be. Approximately two thirds of your immune system lies within the walls of your small intestine. This makes sense because your mouth is the major entry point of foreign material into your body. Your immune cells must analyze everything they come across and determine whether it is safe or not.

If your intestinal lining has become more permeable than it should be, large molecules can pass through your intestinal lining where ordinarily they should not be allowed to do that. This greatly increases the workload of the immune system in your intestines. If your gut is leaky, bacteria, bacterial toxins, incompletely digested foods and waste products can all pass through your gut lining and pose a major challenge to your immune system. This greatly increases levels of inflammation in your body and predisposes you to autoimmune disease.

Unfortunately modern living promotes leaky gut syndrome. The following factors all promote the condition:

• Stress
• Sugar consumption
• Alcohol
• Non-steroidal anti-inflammatory drugs such as aspirin, ibuprofen and naproxen
• Food allergy and intolerance
• Gluten intolerance
• Dysbiosis (too much bad bacteria, not enough good bacteria in the intestines)
• Constipation
• Antibiotics
• The oral contraceptive pill

Avoiding those substances helps to repair leaky gut syndrome. It is also essential to adopt an anti-inflammatory diet, and certain supplements help to repair the gut lining. The most important supplements are a probiotic, glutamine, fish oil, selenium and vitamin D. Their benefits are explained later in this chapter. It is vital to repair a leaky gut in order to improve immune function, reduce inflammation and address immune mediated infertility.

Treatment plan for immune system mediated infertility

As we have mentioned, excess inflammation is endemic in the Western world and this has a detrimental effect on the health of your immune system and reproductive system. Therefore every couple struggling with infertility would greatly benefit from following the recommendations on the next few pages. However, if you fall into one of the categories below, it is essential you follow our anti-inflammatory plan:

- Have been diagnosed with one or more autoimmune diseases.
- You have been diagnosed with endometriosis, or you suffer with the symptoms of endometriosis, particularly painful menstrual periods
- If you know you have several allergies to either foods, or airborne substances or medication.
- If you have at least four symptoms from the allergy list on page 82 but have not been formally diagnosed with allergies

Essential nutrients for reducing inflammation and improving immune function

Supplementing with the following nutrients can help couples with immune system problems to conceive, and these nutrients can often overcome so-called unexplained infertility. These nutrients are vital for anyone with auto-antibodies that are interfering with conception or causing repeat miscarriage. This could be thyroid antibodies, lupus antibodies, anti-phospholipid antibodies, anti-sperm antibodies and others.

Vitamin D

This vitamin has a starring role in the prevention and treatment of autoimmune disease and inflammation. Vitamin D is far more than just a vitamin; it is actually a hormone precursor and regulates the activity of more than 1000 genes in the human body. You would be well aware that vitamin D is required for strong bones, and deficiency leads to osteoporosis, but this vitamin has many more vital functions in the body. Vitamin

D gets manufactured in your skin when you are exposed to sunshine. Specifically it is UVB rays that stimulate the cholesterol in your skin to be converted into a pre-vitamin D substance. The manufacture of vitamin D is then completed in your liver and kidneys.

Most people with indoor lifestyles do not have optimal vitamin D blood levels. The sun's UVB rays are only present during the middle of the day; a time when most people are indoors working. It is important to avoid becoming sunburnt, but regular brief exposure to midday sunshine can have enormously beneficial effects on your health by boosting your vitamin D status. Very few foods provide much vitamin D; egg yolks and oily fish are the best source.

The following individuals are most at risk of vitamin D deficiency:

- Dark skinned individuals
- People covered extensively by clothing or veils
- Anyone who spends most of their time indoors
- People with digestive disorders that impair nutrient absorption. For example celiac disease or inflammatory bowel disease
- People with chronic kidney or liver disease
- The further away you live from the equator, the more likely you are to be vitamin D deficient.
- People living in areas with high levels of air pollution. This reduces the ability of UVB rays to penetrate the earth.
- Anyone who wears sunscreen every time they go outdoors
- People who follow a very low fat diet
- People taking certain medication; for example drugs for epilepsy and cholesterol lowering drugs. Ironically prednisone, which is commonly used for autoimmune disease interferes with vitamin D activation in the body.
- Overweight people are usually vitamin D deficient. This is because vitamin D is fat soluble, so it accumulates in their body fat, rather than in the bloodstream where it is needed.

Why is vitamin D important?

Vitamin D acts as an immune modulator in the body; that means it helps to balance the immune system. Your white blood cells contain vitamin D receptors and require adequate vitamin D for their function. Vitamin D is a powerful natural anti-inflammatory. It helps to reduce excessive production of inflammatory chemicals in your body called cytokines. Vitamin D deficiency is a major trigger of autoimmune disease in genetically susceptible individuals. Vitamin D helps to suppress excess T helper 1 cell activity and it stimulates the production of T regulatory cells. This is a necessary adjustment in order to allow implantation of an embryo and a healthy pregnancy. Excess T helper 1 cell activity and reduced T regulatory cell activity increase the risk of infertility, miscarriage, pre-eclampsia and pre-term delivery. Adequate vitamin D is also vitally important to help your body fight infections. Vitamin D deficiency increases the risk of overgrowth of unfavorable bacteria in the vagina and cervix.

How to know if you are vitamin D deficient

You may hear various recommendations on the length of time you should spend in the sun each week in order to obtain sufficient vitamin D. Such recommendations are not helpful because everyone is an individual and their skin tone, state of health, where they live and a plethora of other factors determine how much vitamin D their skin is able to manufacture. The only way to know if you have enough vitamin D in your bloodstream is through a blood test. Your level of 25 OH vitamin D should be between 100 and 150 nmol/L (40 to 60 ng/mL).

The pathology company that performed the blood test will probably state that a level above 51 nmol/L is sufficient but your vitamin D level should be far higher for optimum health. For most people it is impractical to spend the amount of time in the sun required to manufacture sufficient vitamin D, therefore a vitamin D supplement is essential. It will usually take a couple of months to achieve the desired blood level.

Selenium

Selenium is a trace mineral that has many vital functions in your body. Selenium is incorporated into a number of proteins inside your body, called selenoproteins, that act as powerful antioxidants. Selenium has an anti-inflammatory effect in your body by mopping up free radicals that cause wear and tear to your tissues. Selenium is required for the production of the powerful antioxidant called glutathione peroxidase. This substance is made in your liver and helps to detoxify your body from harmful substances. A low level of antioxidants in the body has been shown to correlate with autoimmune disease flare ups; this has been well studied in patients with lupus.[36]

There is a strong association between autoimmune thyroid disease and selenium deficiency. Selenium deficiency can trigger the disease and hasten its progress. Research has shown that taking a selenium supplement of 200 micrograms per day can reduce blood levels of thyroid antibodies back to normal.[37] The presence of thyroid antibodies in the bloodstream is strongly linked with infertility; therefore a selenium supplement is vital. Selenium is also essential for the production of active thyroid hormone. Thyroid hormone production needs to greatly increase during pregnancy, to provide for the developing fetus before its thyroid gland is formed. Many women cannot produce sufficient thyroid hormone while they are pregnant; therefore a selenium supplement is very important.

Every woman and man with any autoimmune disease, allergies, or excess inflammation needs to take a selenium supplement. It is impossible to obtain enough selenium from food as very few foods are a good source of this mineral. Brazil nuts are usually a good source of selenium but that depends on the quality of the soil in which they were grown. The best absorbed form of selenium in supplements is selenomethionine. This is referred to as organic selenium because it is bound to the amino acid methionine. An ideal daily dose of selenium is 200 micrograms.

Vitamin C

Vitamin C helps to dampen down excess inflammation because it is a powerful antioxidant. Vitamin C supplementation improves autoimmune disease and allergies. It is almost impossible to obtain enough vitamin C through diet alone. You would have to grow your own fruit and vegetables and live in a pollution free and stress free environment. We use up huge quantities of vitamin C when we are exposed to toxins, pollution and when we are stressed. In fact the majority of vitamin C in your body is in your adrenal glands. An ideal dose of vitamin C is between three and six grams a day. It is best taken in divided doses because if you take too much vitamin C at once it can have a laxative effect.

Probiotics

Probiotics are good bowel bacteria, such as acidophilus, bifidus and others. We all have approximately three kilograms of bacteria inside our intestines. We have ten times more bacterial cells in and on our body than we have human cells. Therefore the strains and quantity of bacteria in your digestive tract has an enormous bearing on your health. Good bacteria are strongly anti-inflammatory, whereas bad bacteria secrete highly inflammatory substances. Certain strains of gram negative bacteria inside your digestive tract produce a highly inflammatory substance called lipopolysaccharide. It is one of the most toxic and destructive substances in your body. Therefore, having high levels of bad gut bacteria puts an enormous strain on your immune system and hugely increases the amount of inflammation and tissue destruction occurring in your body.

Dysbiosis is the term given to describe too much bad bacteria and not enough good bacteria inside the digestive tract. If you are wondering what causes this disruption in bowel flora, the answer is pretty much everything common to the Western diet and lifestyle.

Factors that increase levels of pathological bowel bacteria include:

- Stress
- Sugar consumption
- Certain medication – including antibiotics, steroids, anti-inflammatory drugs, antacids and oral contraceptives
- Alcohol
- Food intolerance and allergy

A good probiotic supplement will help to correct the imbalance of bacteria in your intestines and will do wonders to reduce inflammation and help your immune system. It will help to heal a leaky gut. Eating yoghurt is not an effective way to take a probiotic. In order to get the right quantity and the right strains of bacteria, you will need to take a supplement in capsule or powder form.

Benefits of probiotics to the immune system include:

- Digesting and absorbing certain types of fiber, starches and sugars. The friendly bacteria in your digestive tract convert these substances into a source of energy and various acids which help to keep the bowel walls healthy. Food for good bacteria is called a prebiotic. Prebiotics are predominantly the un-digestible fiber in certain vegetables and fruit. Jerusalem artichoke is a particularly rich source of prebiotics. This vegetable is in season during winter. Eating it will greatly increase the levels of good bugs in your bowel.

- Producing vitamins, absorbing minerals and eliminating toxins. Probiotics manufacture some vitamin K and improve your ability to absorb minerals. They also aid in the metabolism and the breakdown of toxins. This is beneficial because it means your liver will have to do less work breaking down toxic substances. Good bacteria produce short chain fatty acids, which are associated with lower levels of allergies and inflammation.

- Keeping bad bacteria under control. The helpful bacteria produce a substance that kills harmful microbes. It is also literally a competition for space inside your digestive tract; the more good bacteria you have, the less room will be available for bad bacteria.

- Preventing allergies. Good bacteria teach your immune system to distinguish between disease causing microbes and non-harmful antigens (such as foods), and to respond appropriately. This helps to prevent your immune system from overreacting to harmless substances such as foods and pollen, thereby reducing your risk of allergies. An enormous amount of research has shown that improving the composition of bacteria in your bowel greatly reduces your risk of eczema, asthma, hay fever, sinusitis and other allergic conditions.

• Supporting the immune cells inside your digestive tract. The vast majority of immune cells inside your body are in your digestive tract. Good bacteria play a crucial role in the development and operation of the immune system in your digestive tract. They also help your immune cells to produce antibodies against disease causing microbes. Probiotics are beneficial for T regulatory cells, which are white blood cells that regulate the immune system and prevent excessive inflammation.

• Reduce the risk of vaginal infections. The composition of flora in your bowel directly determines the composition of your vaginal flora. Probiotics reduce the risk of bacterial vaginosis.

Glutamine

Glutamine is an amino acid (building block of protein). It is the most abundant free amino acid in the body. Glutamine is the major source of fuel for the cells that line your digestive tract; therefore it is essential for maintaining structural integrity of your digestive lining. It helps to heal a leaky gut. This takes a strain off your immune system and liver. Glutamine helps to make your digestive lining a stronger and healthier barrier. Glutamine is available in powder or capsule form. An ideal dose is two grams twice daily.

6. Genitourinary infections and infertility

Infections of the reproductive tract are a common cause of infertility in women and men, but particularly women. In women, infections are capable of causing inflammation and damage to the pelvic organs, particularly the fallopian tubes. In men infections of the testes or epididymis can result in infertility. A number of different organisms are capable of causing infections and the majority of infections are sexually transmitted. One of the reasons that infections often do more harm to a woman's fertility is because many of them are asymptomatic. A woman doesn't know she is infected, therefore the infection is allowed to wreck havoc on her reproductive organs and she only finds out there is a problem too late. Most of these infections don't only compromise fertility; they can also cause a range of adverse pregnancy outcomes and put the fetus at risk.

Types of infections that can affect fertility

Chlamydia

Chlamydia is the most prevalent sexually transmitted bacterial infection in the world. In Australia there were more than 61 thousand cases reported in 2009.[38] The incidence has quadrupled in the last ten years. In the USA there were 1,244,180 reported cases of chlamydia in 2009. 70 percent of infected women do not get symptoms; the figure is 50 percent among men.[39] Chlamydia infection is the leading cause of ectopic pregnancy, because of damage caused to the fallopian tubes.

In the majority of cases chlamydia does not produce symptoms in women. Some women will experience a vaginal discharge between one and three weeks after contracting the infection. This is usually the only symptom, and it may be mild and ignored. Chlamydia usually causes a urethral discharge in men. In women chlamydia causes infection of the cervix and endometrium (lining of the uterus). If left untreated it can then cause inflammation and damage to the fallopian tubes. Untreated chlamydia infection can lead to pelvic inflammatory disease, which may be symptomless or can cause chronic pelvic pain, deep pain during sexual intercourse, a vaginal discharge or burning pain while urinating.

Pelvic inflammatory disease is a fairly common cause of infertility but it is predicted to become a far greater problem in years to come because of the dramatic rise in chlamydia infection among people in their late teens and 20s. Chlamydia infection can increase the risk of miscarriage, ectopic pregnancy and premature delivery. Pregnant women with chlamydia need to deliver via caesarean section because the infant would become infected if it travelled via the birth canal.

Chlamydia is spread via contact with semen or vaginal secretions. In men the infection can lead to inflammation of the urethra, epididymis and prostate gland. Untreated chlamydia infection can also cause a type of arthritis. One study showed that 21 percent of patients with unexplained arthritis had chlamydia infection.[40] Infection can be prevented with condoms. Antibiotics are required for the treatment of chlamydia, but you can also strengthen your immune system using the suggestions at the end of this chapter.

Gonorrhoea is another sexually transmitted infection that can lead to pelvic inflammatory disease and infertility; however it is far less common than chlamydia. Gonorrhoea often doesn't cause symptoms in women, therefore we recommend you are tested for this infection to rule it out as a potential cause of infertility.

Viruses

The two most common viruses that affect fertility and pregnancy outcomes are herpes and cytomegalovirus.

Cytomegalovirus is a common viral infection that produces mild flu-like symptoms in healthy people. The virus is a member of the herpes family, but so is Epstein Barr virus that causes glandular fever, and the chicken pox virus. The virus is spread through coughing, blood, urine, feces and contact with mucous membranes (such as those of the mouth or genitals).

If a pregnant woman in infected, the virus can cause damage

to the developing brain of the fetus. It is particularly risky to be infected in early pregnancy. The baby may develop mental retardation, hearing loss, liver problems, or it may stop growing. Pregnant women must avoid contact with anybody displaying flu-like symptoms to reduce the risk of contracting this infection. Frequent hand washing and basic hygiene will also help.

Genital herpes is an extremely common infection; one in eight Americans carries the infection but not everyone has symptoms. Genital herpes can be caused by either the herpes simplex type 1 or type 2 viruses. The type one virus most commonly causes cold sores on the lips but it can also cause genital sores. Approximately 80 percent of infected people do not realize they have the infection but they can pass it on to others. Genital herpes is transmitted through vaginal, oral and anal sex. Condoms usually do not prevent the spread of infection because the virus is shed from genital skin not covered by a condom. It is possible to catch herpes from a person while they have an outbreak of blisters, but also in between outbreaks, when there are no symptoms. This is because the virus is shed through the skin. Once you have become infected with the herpes virus you cannot get rid of it. The virus will remain in your body, but you can reduce the risk of outbreaks by keeping your immune system strong.

In men infection with herpes can cause a low sperm count. In one study the ejaculates of 100 men without a history of herpes symptoms were analyzed. The herpes virus was detected in 20 percent of samples. Among 76 men with infertility, the herpes virus was detected in 25 percent.[41] In another study the ejaculate of men whose partners suffered with recurrent miscarriage or failed intrauterine insemination was tested for herpes simplex virus. The virus was detected in 65 percent of samples. Normal looking sperm can be infected with the herpes virus, which increases the risk of pregnancy complications and can compromise the health of the embryo.

If a pregnant woman suffers with an outbreak of herpes close to the time of birth, the baby will need to be delivered via caesarean section, to prevent it from becoming infected. Herpes infection in a newborn can lead to damage to the eyes, central nervous system, skin or liver.

Ureaplasma and Mycoplasma infection

These are common sexually transmitted infections and they are often quite resistant to antibiotic treatment. Ureaplasma urealyticum and mycoplasma hominis or genitalium are the most common infections in this category. These infections increase the risk of infertility, recurrent miscarriage, premature delivery and health problems in the newborn. One study found the incidence of ureaplasma and mycoplasma in the semen of infertile men to be 19.2 percent and 15.8 percent respectively. The presence of mycoplasma genitalium is associated with low sperm count and abnormal sperm morphology (shape).[42] Mycoplasma genitalium is frequently present in women with pelvic inflammatory disease, which commonly causes infertility by damaging the fallopian tubes and lining of the uterus.[43]

These infections may cause no symptoms at all, or they can cause a vaginal discharge, painful deep sexual intercourse, burning while urinating or vaginal itching. In men the infection can cause a urethral discharge or painful urination. A cervical swab in women and urethral swab in men can detect these infections. Because these infections are often not entirely eliminated with antibiotics, it is vital for you and your partner to follow our infection fighting recommendations later on in this chapter, as well as our diet guidelines in chapter 8.

Vaginal discharge

Vaginal discharge is a common symptom in women and it can be caused by a variety of factors. It is normal and common to have a small amount of discharge, particularly around the time of ovulation. Glands in the vagina and cervix produce small amounts of fluid to act as lubrication and keep the tissue healthy. Just like in your digestive tract, the lining of your vagina contains plentiful good bacteria, which help to keep the vagina clean and healthy. The bacteria secrete acids, which are vital for maintaining the normal, slightly acidic pH of the vagina. A normal vaginal discharge does not have an odor and it does not cause irritation or itching.

A vaginal discharge that is caused by an infection can have the following Characteristics:

- Increased quantity of discharge
- Itching, irritation or soreness
- Presence of a rash
- Burning or discomfort during urination, which is accompanied by a discharge
- The presence of blood in the discharge
- Odor. This is typically yeasty or fishy
- Painful sexual intercourse
- Change in consistency of the discharge. It may be foamy or thick and curdled
- Change in color of the discharge. It may become white, yellow, green or gray

See your doctor if you have a vaginal discharge with any of these Characteristics. You will need to have a cervical swab taken, which is then analyzed for the presence of microorganisms. Make sure it is a high cervical swab, otherwise the infection may be missed. Vaginal yeast infections are common and they respond well to antimicrobial herbs, as well as our guidelines later in this chapter.

Trichomonas infection is caused by a protozoan called trichomonas vaginalis. It is usually sexually transmitted but it is possible to catch the infection through swimming pools, spas and on toilet seats. Sometimes the infection causes no symptoms at all, but it typically causes a profuse, foamy vaginal discharge that smells fishy. A cervical swab can detect the infection. Trichomonas infection is treated with antibiotics and your partner also needs to be treated, even if he doesn't have any symptoms.

Gardnerella infection can cause a watery vaginal discharge with a fishy odor. Tiny amounts of the gardnerella bacteria are found in the majority of women, but the bacteria can overgrow and cause symptoms if the normally acidic vagina becomes too alkaline. This typically occurs during pregnancy, after giving birth, from exposure to chronic stress, poor diet and nutritional deficiencies. Gardnerella infection during pregnancy slightly increases the risk of pre-term labor. Gardnerella is treated with antibiotics and your partner will also need to be treated, otherwise he would reinfect you the next time you have intercourse.

Bacterial vaginosis is a general term used to describe a bacterial infection of the vagina. These infections increase the risk of adverse pregnancy outcomes, particularly pre-term labor. Antibiotics are used to treat these infections; most commonly Flagyl (metronidazole). However probiotics (beneficial bacteria like acidophilus) and vitamin D can help to prevent these infections. Research has found that vitamin D deficient women are at greater risk of contracting bacterial vaginosis, because vitamin D deficiency weakens the immune system. A study of 469 women published in the Journal of Nutrition found that those with a blood vitamin D level below 20 nmol/L (8 ng/mL) were 34 percent more prone to bacterial vaginosis than women with a vitamin D level above 80 nmol/L (32ng/mL).[44]

A blood vitamin D level below 20 nmol/L (8 ng/mL) indicates severe vitamin D deficiency and this greatly compromises the health of the immune system. For optimum health we recommend your blood vitamin D level is between 100 and 150 nmol/L (40 to 60 ng/mL).

Thrush

Thrush is an infection caused by the yeast Candida. It is normal for small amounts of Candida to live in your gastrointestinal tract, and mucous membranes, including your vagina. However, if your immune system is weak and your digestive health is poor, Candida is allowed to overgrow. Women with thrush have an overgrowth of bad bacteria and yeast in their digestive tract, and they usually eat too much sugar or foods that are rapidly digested into sugar (bread, pasta, breakfast cereals). Food intolerance increases the risk of thrush.

Thrush causes a discharge that is usually white and creamy. It can cause itching, redness and discomfort in and around the vagina. Sometimes symptoms are minor and go away on their own; other times the infection is severe enough to require treatment. Having thrush while you are pregnant will not harm your baby; however it is an indicator that your immune health is poor, and this should be corrected before you fall pregnant. Women with thrush need to follow our diet guidelines in chapter eight.

Diagnosis of genitourinary infections

Several of these infections do not cause symptoms, however they can cause infertility or increase the risk of pregnancy complications if you do manage to fall pregnant. Therefore it is imperative that you are tested for these infections before attempting conception. The various tests required are covered in detail in chapter 10.

Other infections associated with infertility

Mumps

Mumps is a viral infection that causes fever and swollen salivary glands. It was once a common childhood infection, but is not common among children anymore because of widespread use of the mumps vaccination. Most children who contract mumps make a full recovery, but occasionally mumps can cause inflammation of the testes in men. This is more likely if a man contracts the disease in adulthood. The mumps virus can cause damage to the testes and reduce their ability to manufacture sperm. This can cause long term low sperm count even after the infection has subsided. Mumps can also cause inflammation of the ovaries but this is less common.

Periodontal disease

Periodontal disease is an infection of the gums. It is an indicator of a weakened immune system. The infection can be quite harmful if present while a woman is pregnant. Pregnant women with periodontal disease are seven times more likely to have a premature baby or underweight baby. The risk is increased even further if the infection worsens during pregnancy.[45] It is thought that bacteria in the gums release toxins which travel throughout the bloodstream and adversely affect the fetus.

Periodontal disease includes gingivitis and periodontitis. It is caused by an overgrowth of bacteria on and between the teeth and gums that secrete plaque. If left untreated it can lead to loose teeth and eventual tooth loss. Periodontal disease is most common in people over the age of 50, but it is increasingly seen in people in their 20s and 30s. Brushing and flossing your teeth twice a day reduces your risk of infection because it keeps plaque at bay, but metabolic factors also make you more prone to infection.

The following factors increase the risk of periodontal disease:

Diabetes

Diabetics have high blood sugar and sugar feeds bacteria. Therefore diabetics are more prone to nearly every infection. If you have diabetes, try to get your blood sugar as close to normal as possible; normal is less than 99 mg/dL (5.5 mmol/L). See our book *Diabetes Type 2: You can Reverse it Naturally.*

Cigarette smoking

Smokers are far more likely to develop periodontal disease than non-smokers. Smoking suppresses the immune system and uses up huge quantities of antioxidants in your body, as your body attempts to neutralize the toxins in cigarettes. Most smokers are vitamin C deficient and you need vitamin C for strong and healthy gums. Bleeding gums and gum infections are a classic symptom of vitamin C deficiency.

Poor diet and high stress levels

Stress weakens your immune system and makes you more prone to all types of infections. Diets high in sugar and refined carbohydrates such as white bread, pasta, cakes and biscuits increase the risk of periodontal disease. People who consume a lot of those foods tend to consume very few vegetables; lack of fruit and vegetables in the diet promotes gum infections.

Vitamin D deficiency

This increases the risk of gum infections because it weakens your immune system.

Some medication

Steroids, anti-depressants, oral contraceptives and some heart medication all increase the risk of periodontal disease.[46]

Grinding your teeth

People who grind their teeth in their sleep are at increased risk.

Colds and flu in pregnant women

Pregnant women are at increased risk of catching a cold or flu and they can suffer a more severe infection than non-pregnant women. During pregnancy your immune system is suppressed somewhat. That is a good thing because it prevents your body from destroying the developing embryo inside your uterus. Half of the DNA that makes up the embryo does not belong to you; it belongs to your partner. Therefore your immune system must develop tolerance in order to maintain the pregnancy. Unfortunately this same mechanism makes your immune system less capable of fighting off bacterial and viral infections. Therefore it is critical that your immune system is in peak condition now, before you fall pregnant.

How to reduce your risk of infections and strengthen your immune system

It is impossible to protect yourself from coming into contact with every single bug, but there are several ways to minimize your risk of exposure. It is important to remember that your nutritional status greatly influences how your immune system will cope if you do develop an infection. If you are deficient in important nutrients, you are more likely to develop an infection, and the infection will usually be more severe and longer lasting.

The following tips will help to protect you against infections:

- Good hygiene will prevent you from coming into contact with a lot of infections. Wash your hands regularly; particularly after using the toilet, handling money and using public transport. Wash your hands before handling food. Try not to touch your face too much, particularly your mouth and eyes. This can help prevent colds and flu.
- Practice safe sex. See your doctor to be tested for sexually transmitted infections before and after having sex with a new partner, and ask your partner to be tested as well. Condoms are effective at preventing STIs when used correctly, but they do not prevent the transmission of genital herpes.
- Urinate after sex, in order to wash away bacteria that may lead to a vaginal infection. Make sure you wipe from front to back after having a bowel movement.

• Try to get plenty of sleep and rest. Lack of these compromises the health of your immune system greatly.
• Exercise regularly. Exercise boosts circulation and boosts your immune system. Extremely strenuous exercise, such as that performed by athletes suppresses immune function and makes athletes more susceptible to infections. Moderate exercise boosts immune function.
• Follow a healthy diet. Sugar and refined carbohydrates weaken your immune system and make you more prone to infections. Adequate protein is vital for healthy immunity, as are vegetables and fruits. Follow our diet recommendations in chapter 8.
• Ensure you are not deficient in the key nutrients vital for a strong immune system. These nutrients are:
• **Selenium.** Selenium is a mineral that is deficient in the soil of many parts of the world. Selenium reduces your risk of catching infections, and it helps your immune cells to overcome an infection you do have. Selenium reduces the ability of viruses to replicate in your body. People who are selenium deficient tend to get a worse case of a viral infection than people who aren't deficient. Selenium also helps to reduce inflammation, which is a consequence of infections or autoimmune disorders. The best form of selenium to take in supplements is called selenomethionine. An ideal dose is 200 micrograms per day. A blood test is not a useful way to check for selenium deficiency. Clinical trials often assess a person's selenium status via analyzing toenail clippings, but this test is not available to the general public.
• **Zinc.** Zinc deficiency is extremely common. An Australian study found that 85 percent of women and 65 percent of men do not consume the recommended daily intake of zinc.[47] Zinc is very important for hormone production and sperm production, but it also strengthens your immune system and makes you less prone to infections. A low white blood cell count is a common finding in a blood test and zinc deficiency is often the culprit. Zinc deficiency greatly increases your risk of Candida yeast infection.[48] The recommended intake of zinc in supplement form is between 20 and 40 milligrams per day.

- **Vitamin C**. Vitamin C is a water soluble vitamin; therefore your body can't store it. Vitamin C is required for a strong and healthy immune system and fights viruses by inhibiting their ability to replicate. It does this by inhibiting a protein called neuraminidase, which viruses use to duplicate themselves. Severe vitamin C deficiency is called scurvy and it is rare; however mild vitamin C deficiency is incredibly common. Smokers and people who don't eat a lot of fruit and vegetables are most at risk of deficiency.

  Symptoms of vitamin C deficiency include nose bleeds, depression, fatigue, rough and dry skin and poor wound healing. The recommended daily intake of vitamin C is only 30 mg for women and 40 mg for men, but that is a quantity to prevent scurvy, not a quantity necessary to achieve optimum health. Two-time Nobel laureate Linus Pauling suggested that the RDI of vitamin C should be increased to 200mg per day.[49] Modern diets and lifestyles increase vitamin C requirements way beyond that level. A beneficial dose is between 2 and 4 grams of vitamin C per day. It is best taken in divided doses.

- **Vitamin D**. Until recently, no one suspected that vitamin D had functions in our body besides calcium absorption and bone strength. However in recent years vitamin D's significant role in immune health has been discovered. Vitamin D deficiency makes you more prone to all types of infections and greatly impairs your body's ability to overcome infections. Most people require a vitamin D supplement, as they do not spend enough time outdoors to manufacture sufficient quantities of this vitamin through sunlight exposure.

7. Miscarriage

A miscarriage is a devastating event for any couple, but is particularly difficult for couples struggling with long term infertility. Miscarriages are very common; it is thought that approximately 25 percent of known pregnancies result in miscarriage. In many cases a miscarriage occurs in the earliest stages of pregnancy, before a woman even realizes she is pregnant. Experts estimate that between 30 and 50 percent of all pregnancies result in miscarriage. Despite this fact, the vast majority of women who have experienced a miscarriage will go on to have a successful pregnancy. Less than five percent of women experience two consecutive miscarriages, and only one percent experience three or more.[50] Most miscarriages occur in the first 12 weeks of pregnancy.

Symptoms of miscarriage

The biggest indicator of impending miscarriage is vaginal bleeding, although fortunately not all cases of bleeding during pregnancy result in miscarriage. Roughly half of pregnancies with early vaginal bleeding go to full term and produce a healthy baby.

The most common symptoms of miscarriage include:

- Vaginal bleeding - can include brown spotting, light or heavy bleeding
- Lower abdominal cramps
- Severe or sudden back ache
- Fainting
- Excessive nausea or vomiting
- Fever
- Joint pain
- Extreme fatigue
- A gush of clear fluid from the vagina
- Dizziness

Sometimes the fetal tissue and entire placenta are passed out of the body, but oftentimes some tissue will remain inside the uterus. It is very important to see your doctor if you have miscarried, because you will probably need a D and C (dilation and curettage) performed in order to remove all of the tissue from the pregnancy. If tissue is left behind, this could cause a serious infection. The fetal tissue should be analyzed by a laboratory to try and determine the cause of the miscarriage.

Causes of miscarriage

There are several well known factors that can cause miscarriage, and they will be explained on the following pages. In some cases of recurrent miscarriage, doctors cannot determine a cause and therefore between 50 and 75 percent of miscarriage is labeled unexplained. We believe nutritional and immune system factors are responsible for the majority of these cases and this will be explained in the section that follows.

Miscarriage is usually a result of one or more of the following factors:

Genetic/chromosomal causes

Chromosomal abnormalities are said to account for approximately 50 to 70 percent of miscarriages, and this typically occurs in the first pregnancy. Chromosomes are tiny thread-like structures found in the centre of your cells. Your cells contain 46 chromosomes, which are arranged into 23 pairs. One chromosome of the pair came from your mother, and the other came from your father. Chromosomes consist of DNA and they determine your physical attributes such as hair and eye color, as well as physical functions in your body.

Sperm and eggs only contain 23 chromosomes, therefore when they come together at conception, the baby receives 46 chromosomes. When the sperm and egg join at conception, the one cell is called a zygote. It rapidly divides as it grows into a baby. Sometimes the cell splits unevenly and therefore a cell ends up with an incorrect number of chromosomes. The fetus cannot develop properly and a miscarriage occurs. Sometimes these genetic abnormalities can be a result of exposure of the eggs, sperm or developing embryo to environmental chemicals, radiation, or to nutritional deficiencies.

Approximately five percent of couples experience a miscarriage due to an inherited chromosomal rearrangement. Translocation and inversion are the most common inherited chromosomal abnormalities. This is where part of one chromosome is attached to another chromosome or where a segment of a chromosome is reversed. The parent who carries this abnormality is usually normal and unaware of their problem, however their embryo may receive too little or too much genetic material when they attempt to have children. Couples with translocations, inversions and other specific chromosomal abnormalities may need to resort to IVF, with the use of pre-implantation genetic diagnosis.

A mutation of the gene MTHFR can impair your body's ability to use folic acid. This mutation affects approximately 25 percent of the population and some studies have shown it increases the risk of miscarriage. There is more information about this gene on page 188.

Age

The risk of miscarriage increases as men and women get older. In women the risk begins to increase slowly at 27 years of age. 35 year old women have a 25 percent risk of having a miscarriage, and women over 40 have a 33 percent increased risk. The closer a woman is to menopause, the poorer quality eggs she has and the more likely chromosomal abnormalities become. It is well known that the risk of Down syndrome is high in women over the age of 35, but all other less well known genetic abnormalities are also more common. Therefore a miscarriage is a protective mechanism in a pregnancy that would not produce a healthy child.

All of the eggs inside your ovaries were formed three months before you were born. The longer you live, the more environmental chemicals you are exposed to; the more free radical damage occurs to your cells and the greater the risk of genetic defects in your cells. This increases your risk of cancer as you get older but it also increases the risk of genetic problems in your eggs and developing embryo in your uterus.

In men, chromosomal abnormalities in sperm increase with advancing age. Sperm from a 50 year old man causes double the amount of miscarriages of sperm from a 20 year old man.[51]

Older men produce more sperm with genetic abnormalities and motility abnormalities.

Hormonal abnormalities

Adequate progesterone is vital to maintain pregnancy. Progesterone is produced by the corpus luteum after the egg has been released at ovulation. If fertilization occurs, the corpus luteum continues to manufacture progesterone until the placenta has developed and is able to take over progesterone production. Many women are progesterone deficient and they are not able to produce enough progesterone to hold a pregnancy. Inadequate progesterone production is often referred to as luteal phase deficiency or defect and this may cause repeated miscarriage.

Progesterone supplementation is very effective and entirely safe for use in pregnancy in these women. Progesterone supplementation is required for the first 16 weeks of pregnancy; after that the placenta is able to produce sufficient quantities. Sometimes progesterone levels will be low in early pregnancy because the embryo has not implanted in the uterus properly and the pregnancy is not progressing properly. In this instance low progesterone is a symptom of a failed pregnancy, not a cause. In that instance giving supplemental progesterone will usually not help to prevent a miscarriage.

Endometriosis can double the risk of miscarriage. This is due to the chronic inflammation in the lining of the uterus, which creates a hostile environment for the embryo, thus inhibiting proper development. Women with polycystic ovarian syndrome also have higher rates of miscarriage. A number of factors may be responsible for this; women with PCOS often have poorer quality eggs, and the lining of their uterus is less hospitable to implantation by an embryo.

Structural abnormalities

Abnormalities in the structure of the uterus account for approximately ten to 15 percent of recurrent miscarriage. Some women are born with an abnormal uterus (double uterus, uterine septum, or a uterus where only one side has formed). Acquired abnormalities in the uterus include fibroids, polyps, Asherman's syndrome (scar tissue in the uterine cavity). In some instances these abnormalities can be surgically corrected. Cervical incompetence can cause miscarriage after 14 weeks but can be remedied with the insertion of a cervical stitch by a doctor. Cone biopsy, which is a treatment used on women with cervical cancer can weaken the cervix and increase the risk of miscarriage.

Immune system disorders

A number of subtle immune system problems can prevent the progression of a normal pregnancy. These often occur in the very early stages of pregnancy, so a woman may not even realize she was pregnant. It is quite remarkable how the immune system is designed to protect you from foreign substances such as bacteria, viruses and anything that is not self tissue, yet the fetus growing inside the uterus is comprised of 50 percent foreign tissue (the father's DNA) and this is not rejected by your immune cells.

Women with autoimmune disease typically suffer with infertility and repeated miscarriage. Antiphospholipid syndrome is an autoimmune disorder that accounts for three to 15 percent of recurrent miscarriages. The presence of anti-cardiolipin antibodies or lupus anti-coagulant antibodies in the bloodstream can confirm the presence of antiphospholipid syndrome. These blood tests should both be performed again six weeks later for confirmation. Antibodies to phospholipid molecules can cause damage to the inside of blood vessel walls. This allows blood cells to stick to the site of injury and promotes blood clots. Therefore placental blood vessels cannot form properly. Some phospholipid molecules have glue-like properties and allow cells to fuse together. This is a vital process in the formation of the placenta. Antibodies against these molecules interfere with the normal formation of the placenta. This prevents the supply of blood, oxygen and nutrients to the developing embryo, therefore a miscarriage results.

Women with antiphospholipid antibodies who are not able to maintain a pregnancy are treated with a low dose of aspirin (typically 80mg) and the blood thinner heparin (low molecular weight form of heparin called nadroparin). The success of this therapy is increased if a woman starts taking these drugs before conception and continues right through the pregnancy. Some doctors promote the use of aspirin and heparin for all women who have had at least two miscarriages. Research has shown this to be ineffective in many cases. There is only a small group of women who benefit from this therapy, and even women with blood clotting disorders do not always benefit.

Fortunately diet changes and nutritional medicine are extremely effective in the treatment of autoimmune disease and can greatly increase your chance of a healthy full term pregnancy. Every autoimmune disease increases the risk of infertility and miscarriage, including celiac disease, lupus, autoimmune thyroid disease and any condition associated with raised antinuclear antibodies in the bloodstream. These conditions inhibit implantation of the embryo and/or inhibit the proper development of the placenta. See chapter 5 for our recommendations for autoimmune disease.

Sometimes the immune disorder that causes miscarriage is far more subtle. In the earliest stages of pregnancy, the mother's immune system receives chemical signals from the tiny embryo. Some of these signals come from the father's DNA inside the embryo. Some of these messages involve antigens on white blood cells. Your white blood cells contain molecules on their surface called Human Leukocyte Antigens (HLA). These molecules are unique to every individual and they help your body to recognize your own tissues from foreign substances such as microbes, cancer cells, transplanted organs and fetuses.

Half of the HLA molecules inside the embryo are from you and half of them are from the father. When you become pregnant, your immune system recognizes that there are foreign HLA molecules inside your uterus. Therefore in a normal healthy pregnancy, the mother's white blood cells inside her uterus produce substances called blocking antibodies. These ingenious molecules coat the fetal cells and protect them from the mother's natural killer cells. Natural killer cells are a type of white blood cell that is designed to do just as the name suggests; they particularly kill virus infected cells and cancer cells. Sometimes the mother's HLA molecules are too similar to the father's HLA molecules. Therefore the mother's immune system doesn't recognize the difference and does not produce the protective blocking antibodies. Approximately one in every

200 couples is too genetically similar to achieve a successful pregnancy. There are immune therapies available to treat this condition and you can read more on the website www.rialab. com

Abnormally high levels of the type of white blood cells called natural killer cells can result in miscarriage, as these cells can damage the embryo and placenta. An imbalance in T helper cells can also cause miscarriage. T helper cells are a type of white blood cell. There are two major categories of these cells: T helper 1 cells and T helper 2 cells. T helper 1 cells are involved in strong, rapid removal of infectious agents and foreign tissue, whereas T helper 2 cells are far less aggressive. During a normal healthy pregnancy, T helper 2 cells become the dominant cells in the placenta. Some cases of repeated miscarriage are caused by a failure to shift to T helper 2 cells in the placenta.[52] Adequate progesterone production is vital for this immune system shift and administering progesterone to women with recurrent miscarriage can prevent the immune system problems that cause the embryo to be destroyed by the immune system. See page 49 for a more detailed explanation of the benefits of progesterone in autoimmune disease.

Thrombophilia

Thrombophilia means an increased tendency to form blood clots. There are several different conditions that can predispose a woman to increased blood clot formation. Some cases of thrombophilia are genetic and the person is born that way, and other cases are acquired and are a symptom of another disease. Antiphospholipid, anti-cardiolipin and lupus anticoagulant antibodies can all cause thrombophilia. Thrombophilia can increase the risk of fetal death in the earliest stages of pregnancy, right up to the second half of pregnancy.

Blood tests to check how fast your blood clots can be organized. These tests include Prothrombin Time (PT) and Activated Partial Thromboplastin Time (aPTT). You should also be tested for Protein C, Factor V Leiden, Protein S deficiency, Prothrombin gene mutation and Antithrombin III deficiency. Abnormal results are usually an indicator of a hereditary condition.

Metabolic disorders

Poorly controlled diabetes increases the risk of miscarriage. Diabetic women should try to get their blood sugar as close to ideal as possible before conception. Ideal blood sugar is less than 5.5 mmol/L in the fasting state. The drug metformin can reduce the risk of miscarriage in diabetics, however the drug does cause vitamin B 12 deficiency, therefore blood levels of this vitamin should be monitored. Women with syndrome X (insulin resistance) also have a higher rate of miscarriage. Syndrome X is a forerunner to type 2 diabetes. Women with polycystic ovarian syndrome and high blood pressure are at greater risk of miscarriage. Being overweight (BMI above 30) and being underweight (BMI below 19) are both associated with an increased incidence of miscarriage.

Infections

A number of infections in the mother increase the risk of miscarriage; these include chlamydia, mycoplasma, ureaplasma, listeria, toxoplasmosis, bacterial vaginosis, rubella, herpes, measles, mumps, parvovirus and hepatitis A, B or C.

Environmental factors

A great number of environmental chemicals are known to increase the risk of miscarriage, and some occupations are particularly hazardous. Female veterinarians are at double the risk of miscarriage due to exposure to anaesthetic gases and pesticides. An Australian study also showed that female vets who performed more than 5 X rays a week were 80 percent more likely to miscarry than vets performing fewer X rays.[53]

If chemicals and radiation are capable of having such a profound effect on pregnant women, they are surely capable of harming the health of non-pregnant people as well. Radiation is capable of causing DNA damage inside our cells and that is how it increases the risk of cancer. However as we get older, our cells become less susceptible to harm caused by radiation. At no time are you more sensitive to the effects of radiation and environmental chemicals than when you were inside your mother's uterus. The rapidly growing and dividing cells of the embryo are intensely vulnerable to the effects of these substances. For this reason, no pregnant woman should travel in an aeroplane. Flying in the late stages of pregnancy is known to increase the risk of premature labor and all doctors advise women against it. But women should not fly at any stage of pregnancy. In addition to the increased risk of miscarriage, radiation exposure increases the risk of congenital birth defects and childhood cancer.

Electromagnetic radiation also poses a risk. In our modern lives electromagnetic radiation is pervasive and impossible to completely avoid. A great deal of research has linked chronic exposure to strong electromagnetic fields to cancer in humans. A study published in the journal Epidemiology recruited 900 pregnant women and asked them to wear a monitor for 24 hours to measure their level of exposure to electromagnetic radiation. The researchers found that women with the highest exposure had an 80 percent increased risk of miscarriage. The risk was even higher among women with a history of recurrent miscarriage and/or infertility.[54]

Every cell in your body is surrounded by an electromagnetic field, and various parts of your body, such as your brain and other organs have their own electromagnetic field. The weak electromagnetic fields of your body are easily disrupted by the extremely strong electromagnetic fields of modern appliances. Some modern appliances emit much stronger electromagnetic radiation than others; top offenders include electric blankets, hairdryers, radios, refrigerators, irons, blenders, toasters, televisions and of course mobile phones. The good news is the radiation level drops significantly the further away you are from the appliance. With most appliances there is no significant electromagnetic field at one and a half meters. Therefore try to keep your distance from appliances when possible and do not have too many electrical appliances in your bedroom.

Some high risk occupations for miscarriage include hairdressers, nail technicians, dentists and dental nurses, flight attendants and women employed in construction, agriculture, forestry and petrochemicals. Bisphenol A, a chemical found in some types of plastic is linked to a higher risk of miscarriage. Non-steroidal anti-inflammatory drugs like aspirin and ibuprofen can both increase miscarriage risk in some women. Exposure to tobacco smoke, alcohol and caffeine in excess of 300 mg daily all increase the risk and this topic is covered in more detail in chapter 8

Some antidepressant medication increases the risk of miscarriage and adverse fetal outcomes. A study published in the Canadian Medical Association Journal showed a 68 percent increased risk of miscarriage among women taking prescription antidepressants. Researchers analyzed data on 5,124 women in Quebec and found the risk was highest for selective serotonin reuptake inhibitors (SSRIs) and serotonin-noradrenaline reuptake inhibitors; in particular paroxetine (Paxil, Aropax) and venlafaxine (Efexor).[55]

Nutrient deficiencies

Poor diet and nutritional deficiencies in the mother and father increase the risk of miscarriage. The most important nutrients are selenium, B vitamins (including folic acid), vitamin D, zinc, magnesium, manganese, essential fatty acids, vitamin A and vitamin E.

Male factors

Increasing evidence has shown that abnormalities in sperm can have adverse effects on embryo development and miscarriage risk. Men with low sperm counts have a higher incidence of miscarriage. When the sperm count is low, the quality of the sperm is suboptimal as well. High levels of DNA fragmentation inside the sperm are linked to a range of adverse pregnancy outcomes. This topic is covered in detail in chapter 11.

Stress

High levels of stress in a woman increases the risk of miscarriage. When you are stressed, your brain releases a hormone called corticotropin releasing hormone (CRH). Women who go into premature labor or have low birth weight infants are usually found to have high levels of this hormone in their bloodstream. It is interesting to note that the placenta also releases corticotropin releasing hormone at the time of labor to stimulate uterine contractions during delivery. CRH has a powerful effect on mast cells, which are a type of white blood cell. Mast cells are typically associated with allergic reactions but these cells are abundant in the placenta. Researchers believe that CRH stimulates mast cells of the placenta to secrete an enzyme that destroys tissue, thereby triggering a miscarriage. Women with recurrent miscarriages are found to have high levels of CRH in their placenta. [56]. Stress has terribly destructive effects on our bodies and it is vital to try and minimize it any way you can.

Thyroid disorders

Autoimmune thyroid disease increases the risk of miscarriage. Women who test positive for thyroid antibodies in their bloodstream are at increased risk of infertility, miscarriage, IVF failure, fetal death, pre-eclampsia, premature delivery, postpartum thyroiditis and postnatal depression.[57] Even women who do not have autoimmune thyroid disease and do not have thyroid antibodies are at increased risk of miscarriage if their TSH level is not in the optimum range. Thyroid Stimulating Hormone (TSH) is made by the pituitary gland in the brain and it stimulates your thyroid gland to manufacture appropriate amounts of hormones. If TSH becomes elevated it means your thyroid gland is unable to produce sufficient quantities of hormones. This may be due to immune system disorders, nutrient deficiencies or environmental factors.

Recent research has shown that even women with high supposedly "normal" TSH levels are at increased risk of miscarriage. The results of a recent study were presented at the Endocrine Society 92nd Annual Meeting in San Diego. The study looked at 4 000 women who tested negative for thyroid antibodies and had a TSH of 5.0 or lower at nine weeks into their pregnancy. Researchers found that the rate of miscarriage was 6.1 percent in women with a TSH between 2.5 and 5.0 mIU/L and 3.6 percent among women with a TSH below 2.5 mIU/L. Therefore a TSH level in the upper half of "normal" almost doubles the risk of miscarriage.[58]

Back in 2007 an Endocrine Society committee recommended that TSH should be no higher than 2.5 in the first trimester of pregnancy, and no higher than 3 in the second and third trimesters. It is normal for TSH to rise slightly in pregnancy because your thyroid gland has to cope with a greatly increased workload as your baby grows.

The take home message is to make sure you have a thyroid blood test while trying to conceive and regularly throughout your pregnancy. Don't be satisfied with your doctor telling you your hormone levels are normal, because "normal" means different things to different doctors. What you need is optimal thyroid hormone levels and if you are trying to conceive, your TSH should be between 0.3 and 2.5 mIU/L.

Natural ways to reduce the risk of miscarriage

Along with awareness of the risk factors for miscarriage discussed in the previous pages, the following nutritional strategies can greatly help reduce the risk:

You and your partner need to be in the best possible health. For three to six months before attempting to conceive, you must pay particular attention to your diet and lifestyle. Both of you need to follow the anti-inflammatory diet described in chapter 8. Your diet and lifestyle are just as important before you become pregnant as during your pregnancy.

- Supplement with folic acid and vitamin B12.
- Selenium can greatly reduce the risk of miscarriage.
- Ensure you receive adequate zinc
- Supplement with omega 3 essential fatty acids
- Supplement with vitamin D
- Make sure you are not zinc deficient

See page 144 for recommended doses of these nutrients.

Case study: recurrent miscarriage

Lisa came to see me desperately wanting to have a second child. She already had a three year old son, who she conceived with the help of Clomid and intrauterine insemination (IUI). Lisa had a long history of infertility. She was 34 when she had her son and had been trying to conceive for two years. Lisa had an irregular menstrual cycle that varied in length between 28 and 42 days. She was always a slim girl and worked as a fitness instructor, yet she had symptoms of polycystic ovarian syndrome (PCOS). No doctor actually investigated Lisa for PCOS though. Because of her irregular cycle and inability to conceive, it was assumed she was not ovulating regularly and she was given Clomid.

When her son was two years old Lisa tried to have a second child. She did manage to conceive after only four months of trying but had a miscarriage at eight weeks. Six months later

Lisa had another miscarriage at nine weeks. Lisa did not want to use Clomid again, and she wanted to know if there was a way to prevent her suffering with another miscarriage. No doctor investigated the reason for her two miscarriages and Lisa wanted to first concentrate on improving her state of health, before undergoing any investigations.

Lisa was slim and fit when she came to me but she suffered with a lot of abdominal bloating. By the end of the day she felt extremely uncomfortable, and she often suffered with bouts of diarrhea for no known reason. Lisa also often had blocked sinuses and a blocked nose at night. Her cholesterol and triglycerides were surprisingly high for someone so slim and fit. This is often the case in women with PCOS.

I put Lisa on a low carbohydrate eating plan, as outlined on page 40 She had previously eaten a great deal of flour based foods, and thought she could get away with it because she wasn't overweight. I also put Lisa on a gluten and dairy free diet. This completely cleared her blocked nose and sinuses and completely eliminated the abdominal bloating and diarrhea, which Lisa was thrilled about.

I gave Lisa the following supplements:

Vitamin D - 2000 IU daily

Iodine - 320 mcg

Zinc – 30 mg

Selenium 200 mcg

Lisa managed to convince her husband to take those supplements as well. I also gave Lisa a probiotic and fish oil. Lisa was given a progesterone cream and told to use one gram each evening.

I saw Lisa twice over three months and we discussed her meal plan and supplements. 13 weeks after Lisa's initial consultation, she phoned me to tell me she was pregnant. She and her husband were extremely excited but also quite apprehensive and didn't want to get their hopes up too high. Fortunately Lisa had a comfortable and healthy pregnancy and gave birth to a healthy baby girl who arrived two days early.

Lisa achieved success unusually quickly and I believe it was largely due to her high level of motivation to follow my diet and supplement recommendations to the letter. When Lisa rang me to tell me she was pregnant, she commented that she had never felt healthier in her life, and because of that she strongly believed that this pregnancy would go to term.

Although recurrent miscarriage is a devastating experience; it is important to remember that the majority of couples will go on to achieve a healthy pregnancy and baby.

Preventing pre-eclampsia and eclampsia

Pre-eclampsia is a pregnancy induced disease associated with high blood pressure and the presence of protein in the urine during the second half of pregnancy. Women typically experience a rapid rise in weight and extreme swelling of their hands, feet and face. Pre-eclampsia is a fairly common condition that affects approximately eight percent of pregnancies. Pre-eclampsia may even occur up to six weeks post-partum but this is not common. The term eclampsia refers to epileptic seizures during pregnancy; it occurs if pre-eclampsia is not treated. Eclampsia is very rare in developed nations; it tends to occur mainly in developing nations where there is poor access to medical care.

Factors that increase the risk of pre-eclampsia

- The risk is highest with the first pregnancy.
- Very young mothers (teenagers) and women over the age of 35 are at increased risk
- Multiple pregnancy - with twins, triplets or more
- Having a family history of pre-eclampsia or experiencing pre-eclampsia in a previous pregnancy
- Pregnancy with a new sexual partner. The longer a couple have been having sex, the lower the risk of pre-eclampsia. A sexual relationship of less than four months duration increases the risk.[59]
- Obesity
- Diabetes
- High blood pressure and/or kidney disease

- Thyroid disease
- Sleep deprivation. Getting less than five hours of sleep per night during pregnancy increases the risk.
- Autoimmune disease
- Vitamin D deficiency
- Selenium deficiency
- Co enzyme Q10 deficiency
- Magnesium deficiency. Taking 400 mg of magnesium in supplement form greatly reduces the risk of developing pre-eclampsia. It is easiest to achieve this dosage with a magnesium powder.
- Dysbiosis. This means having too many bad bugs and not enough good bugs in the digestive tract
- Consumption of trans fatty acids. These are commonly found in processed foods and listed as partially hydrogenated vegetable oil or vegetable fat on food labels.

What causes pre-eclampsia?

Pre-eclampsia occurs when there is a problem with the normal development of the placenta. It is thought that the mother's immune cells interfere with the normal development of the placenta, and this restricts blood flow through the placenta. The restricted blood flow sends chemical messages through the mother's body that have the effect of severely raising blood pressure. The baby of a pre-eclamptic mother grows more slowly inside the uterus and is at risk of oxygen deficiency. The baby usually has to be delivered prematurely in order to prevent life threatening events to the baby or mother.

A number of theories exist for the etiology of pre-eclampsia but most research indicates that the condition is caused by an immune system disorder in the mother. Research conducted in Sydney and published in the Journal of Immunology confirms that pre-eclampsia is caused by the mother's immune system mounting an attack against the fetus and trying to reject it. The researchers measured the level of a type of white blood cell called T regulatory cells in the blood of healthy pregnant women at the time of delivery and compared them to levels of these cells in women with pre-eclampsia. They found that in healthy women there was an increase in the quantity of T regulatory cells and a reduction in T cells that cause inflammation. Women with pre-eclampsia don't experience this vital shift in immune function during their pregnancy.

Professor Fazekas, lead researcher in this study has stated that "Our research reinforces the belief pre-eclampsia is initiated, at least in part, by an immune mediated problem that leads to an increase in inflammation." He also stated "We found that the changes in the balance between Regulatory T-cells and inflammatory T-cells in pregnancy may be crucial in stopping the mother's immune system from rejecting the baby. In pre-eclampsia, when these changes do not occur, both the baby and the mother are put at risk." [60]

It is also known that the longer a woman is exposed to her partner's sperm and semen, the less likely she is to develop pre-eclampsia. Scientists believe that regular sex with the same man primes a woman's immune system not to reject his sperm when they attempt to conceive. Regular sex for more than four months before attempting to conceive has a protective effect. This obviously means sex where the woman is exposed to semen, as opposed to condom use.

According to doctor Gustaaf Dekker, of the University of Adelaide, Australia, "Eventually when the woman conceives, her immune cells will say "we know that guy, he has been around a long time, we'll allow the pregnancy to continue". After intercourse, a woman's immune system sends cells to the cervix to collect the father's foreign immune system proteins and take them back to the lymph nodes where other immune cells can recognize them. Dr Dekker suggests that semen contains an agent that prompts the woman's immune system to recognize the man's proteins.

Other research has linked regular oral sex with a reduced risk of pre-eclampsia. Approximately 70 to 80 percent of the immune cells in your body live in your gastrointestinal tract. Research published in the Journal of Reproductive Immunology has found that swallowing sperm enables the woman's immune system to tolerate the foreign proteins found in his sperm. Semen contains a type of immune system molecule called Human Leukocyte Antigen (HLA) which identifies the male. [61] So it looks like there are medicinal benefits to swallowing something else along with your vitamin tablets!

Other researchers believe that pre-eclampsia is a distinct autoimmune disease. Biochemists at the University of Texas Medical School at Houston were able to demonstrate that auto antibodies produced in a woman can bind to and activate an angiotensin receptor that results in artery constriction, thereby raising blood pressure and producing pre-eclampsia.

How is pre-eclampsia treated by the medical profession?

Because it can have such serious repercussions, the most common and most effective treatment for pre-eclampsia is delivery of the baby. Pre-eclampsia is a major cause of premature delivery and low birth weight infants. If the infant is too premature and would not survive outside the uterus, a woman is usually given blood pressure medication and told to remain in bed. Lying on the left side is usually recommended as this takes the weight of the baby off the mother's major blood vessels.

How to reduce the risk of pre-term birth (premature labor)

A normal pregnancy lasts approximately 40 weeks. Around 12 percent of pregnancies result in premature labor and this is defined as going into labor before the 37th week. Premature babies are at increased risk of health problems. These include brain and neurological abnormalities, digestive problems and breathing difficulties. Premature babies are at increased risk of developmental delays and learning problems when they start school.

Fortunately there are several well known risk factors for premature labor. Knowing what they are can help you take steps to avoid giving birth prematurely. The following factors increase the risk of premature labor:

- Infections. Sexually transmitted infections, bladder infections and gum infections all increase the risk of premature labor. Get tested for infections before falling pregnant and take steps to strengthen your immune system.
- Diabetes and insulin resistance (syndrome X)
- Being overweight or underweight while pregnant

- Uterine abnormalities, including uterine fibroids
- Women with autoimmune disease are at greater risk. Follow our recommendations for autoimmune disease in chapter 5
- High blood pressure
- Thrombophilia (blood clotting disorder)
- Use of IVF
- Cone biopsy, used in the treatment of cervical dysplasia or cervical cancer
- Vitamin D deficiency
- Zinc deficiency
- Folic acid deficiency
- Stress
- Excess exposure to phthalates. Research has shown that mothers delivering before 37 weeks were found to have up to 10.7 times more phthalate metabolites in their urine.[62]
- Thyroid disease. Follow our recommendations in chapter 3
- Consumption of artificial sweeteners while pregnant increases the risk of pre-term delivery by up to 80 percent. This is thought to be due to the artificial sweetener aspartame.[63] Aspartame is sold commercially as Equal and NutraSweet and listed as food additive number 951 on labels. Make sure you avoid all artificial sweeteners.
- Prolonged periods of standing while pregnant.

Where possible, try to avoid as many of these factors as you can when you are pregnant.

8. Diet and Lifestyle factors affecting fertility

A number of diet and lifestyle conditions have a negative bearing on fertility. The prevalence of these lifestyle factors in society goes a long way towards explaining the escalating incidence of infertility today.

The effect of age on fertility

It is well known that a woman's fertility declines as she ages, but not everyone realizes that the same happens in men. Firstly we'll begin with women. According to an Australian Institute of Health and Welfare study, the average age of Australian women bearing their first child has increased from under 26 years in 1991, to almost 30 years in 2003. By now the age is probably greater than 30. The average age of women undergoing IVF is now 36.5 years. Today one in four women undergoing IVF is 40 years of age or older.

Women are most fertile between the ages of 20 and 24. When a woman reaches 35 years of age her fertility declines dramatically. According to the Human Fertilization and Embryology Authority, at 35 years of age you are half as fertile as when you were 25; by age 40 you are half as fertile as when you were 35. Medically a 35 year old pregnant woman is referred to as an "older mum"; she has the words "advanced maternal age" written on her medical records. If these women do fall pregnant, they have a much higher risk of miscarriage, fetal abnormalities and pregnancy complications. One in six pregnancies leads to a miscarriage in a 30 year old, whereas the risk is one in four in a 40 year old.[64] Down syndrome occurs in 1:1000 pregnancies in a 30 year old woman, but 1:100 pregnancies in a 40 year old. Several other genetic defects are more common in older mums.

Why does fertility decline rapidly in women?

The following factors may be responsible:

- The quality of your ovarian follicles declines. Women do not run out of eggs in their ovaries; hormone levels drop therefore eggs no longer keep developing, and as the body ages the eggs decline in quality.
- Mucus secretions in the vagina and cervix become less hospitable to sperm as women age.
- The endometrial lining can become thinner and less able to allow the impregnation of a fertilized egg.
- Uterine fibroids are more common as women age and they can inhibit fertilization or restrict the growth of an embryo.
- The menstrual cycle can become irregular or shorter. Women with a menstrual cycle of around 30 to 31 days length are the most fertile. The menstrual cycle becomes shorter as women approach menopause.
- The consequences of long term hormonal imbalances have had many years to take effect; for example long term endometriosis can cause scarring and adhesions that inhibit fertility. Pelvic inflammatory disease can also cause long term damage to the reproductive system.
- The likelihood of being exposed to a sexually transmitted infection rises as women get older. Some infections can cause structural damage to the reproductive system.
- Rates of obesity increase as women and men get older. Being overweight or obese can impair fertility.
- Health may decline and chronic diseases may develop as women get older; for example type 2 diabetes or high blood pressure. This will affect fertility.
- The longer you have been alive, the more chemicals have accumulated in your body. Several environmental chemicals are strongly implicated in infertility.

The effects of age on male fertility

Most of us know of several older men who have fathered children. It is possible for some men over the age of 60 to father children, but sperm quality does decline and there are potential risks for the health of the child. Generally most studies have found that potential problems start to surface in fathers over the age of 40. However, a poor diet and an unhealthy lifestyle can cause a man to age much faster and this will affect the quality of his sperm.

A study conducted at Saroka University in Israel analyzed the quality and quantity of the sperm and semen in men of various ages. The study found that semen quality peaked between the ages of 30 and 35, and quality was lowest in men over 55 years. Sperm motility (how well the sperm swim) was best before the age of 25 and lowest after age 55. The quality of the genetic material deteriorates in sperm as men get older and this is a more significant problem. Older men produce sperm with increased levels of DNA fragmentation (DNA damage). Genetic defects in the sperm of older men not only increase the risk of infertility, they also increase the risk of miscarriage and some birth defects. Older men are more likely to pass on genetic problems to their children and there are higher rates of childhood cancer in children with older fathers. Some studies have shown that older men are more likely to have children with lower IQ scores and children with Down syndrome (but only if the mother is over 35).[65]

The most common birth defects that are seen in the children of older fathers include achondroplasia (a type of dwarfism), Marfan syndrome (a connective tissue disorder), neurofibromatosis (causes the growth of benign tumors) and Apert syndrome (causes skull and facial abnormalities). As paternal age increases, so does the frequency of genetic mutations. According to Dr Joe Leigh Simpson, of the American College of Medical Genetics, the risk of sporadic single gene mutations may be four to five times higher for fathers who are 45 years of age or older, compared to fathers in their 20s. Genetic mutations increase the risk of cancer and many other diseases. Even the grandchildren of older fathers are at increased risk of damage to their genes and subsequent diseases.

Rates of autism are higher in the children of older fathers. Men who become fathers at 40 years of age or older are 5.75 times more likely to have a child with autism spectrum disorder than fathers younger than 30. A study conducted in Israel found that the risk of schizophrenia was doubled in children of fathers in their late 40s compared to fathers under 25. The rate increased almost threefold in children born to fathers aged 50 or older. The risk of schizophrenia is one in 99 for fathers aged 30 to 35 and jumps to one in 47 for fathers 50 and older.

As our bodies age, we don't do things as well. The amount of mistakes our cells make during division increases, and that largely explains the increased risk of cancer as we all get older. The ability of men to manufacture sperm cells also declines as they get older. The name given to immature stem cells in the testes that eventually become sperm is spermatogonia. These cells are continually replicating and dividing, with each division increasing the risk of errors. In women, the cells that produce eggs go through approximately 24 divisions; whereas in men the cells that create sperm go through around 30 divisions before puberty and then roughly 23 replications a year from puberty onward. By the time a man is 50 years of age, the cells that create his sperm have been through more than 800 rounds of division and replication. Wherever there is such frequent division of cells, the chance of errors occurring is high. Luckily improvements in diet and lifestyle, as well as certain nutritional supplements can greatly reduce the amount of DNA damage inside sperm cells.

If you or your partner are over the age of 35 you must take extra care of your health to ensure a healthy pregnancy and healthy child. In men and women, the older you are, the more exposure your body has had to environmental chemicals and radiation, and the longer nutritional deficiencies have had their chance to do harm to your body. You will have a higher body burden of chemicals that have had more time to do their damage. If your diet and lifestyle are not ideal, nutritional deficiencies can get worse over time and have more detrimental effects on your body. By following the diet guidelines in this book, and minimizing your exposure to environmental chemicals, you can slow down the ageing process in your body and also extend your number of fertile years.

Obesity

Obese women have more menstrual disturbances, find it more difficult to fall pregnant and have a higher risk of pregnancy and delivery complications. Obesity causes a number of metabolic and hormonal disorders that help to explain these outcomes.

Obese women are more prone to developing insulin resistance (syndrome X). This is especially the case for women who carry excess weight on their abdominal region. Insulin resistance greatly increases the risk of polycystic ovarian syndrome. Women with polycystic ovarian syndrome don't ovulate regularly or at all. Even overweight women who do not have polycystic ovarian syndrome often fail to ovulate, and thus obesity is a major cause of anovulation. Even young obese women who have regular menstrual cycles usually take longer to conceive than slim women.

Obesity causes raised systemic inflammation; therefore overweight women usually have higher levels of an inflammatory marker called C-reactive protein in their bloodstream. In a normal, healthy pregnancy, levels of inflammation in the body increase. Pregnant women have higher numbers of white blood cells called macrophages and neutrophils in their bloodstream, and their level of C-reactive protein increases. A healthy woman's body can compensate for this, but obese women already have inflamed bodies, therefore the increased immune activity is believed to be responsible for many of the complications of pregnancy seen in obese women. Obese women have far less success with IVF and other assisted reproductive technologies than healthy weight women. Losing weight if overweight is one of the fastest ways to achieve a pregnancy.

How to assess your weight

The two most common methods for assessing body weight are body mass index (BMI) and measuring your waist circumference. Body mass index is a measure of body fat based on your height and weight. It isn't perfect because it doesn't account for people with a lot of muscle on their body, but it is a useful rough guide. To determine your BMI you need to divide your weight by your height squared.

Body Mass Index = $\dfrac{\text{WEIGHT (kilograms)}}{\text{HEIGHT X HEIGHT (meters)}}$

For example, if you weigh 75 kilograms and are 1.69 meters tall, your BMI is:

$$\dfrac{75 \text{ kilograms}}{1.69 \times 1.69 \text{ meters}}$$

2.2 kilo = 1 lb
2.5cm = 1 inch
100 cm = 1 meter

BMI = 26

You can use the following scale as a guide:

- Under 18 - very underweight
- Under 20 - underweight
- 20 to 25 - healthy weight range
- 26 to 30 - overweight
- Over 30 - obese

Some would argue that the circumference of your waist is a better indicator of body fat, as excess fat in the abdominal area has the most detrimental health consequences. To measure your waist, do the following:

Use a tape measure and measure yourself directly against your skin. Breathe out normally and make sure the tape is snug, but doesn't compress your skin. Measure your waist roughly in line with your belly button. For most people, a waist measurement higher than the following readings is related to increased health risks:

Increased health risks

Women: greater than 80 centimeters

Men: greater than 94 centimeters

Greatly increased health risks

Women: greater than 88 centimeters

Men: greater than 102 centimeters

Again, these figures are not perfect indicators, as they don't accommodate for all body types. They are most useful for Caucasians; Asians should have even smaller waist measurements for optimum health.

Risks to mother and baby associated with obesity

Being obese while pregnant is associated with a wide range of dangerous health conditions; therefore we strongly urge all obese women to lose weight before attempting to conceive. Maternal obesity is strongly associated with the following:

- Menstrual disorders
- Miscarriage - both early and late stage
- The risk of stillbirth is almost double
- High birth weight infant. Women with high triglycerides (above 150 mg/dL (1.7 mmol/L) are at particular risk of having a large birth weight baby).
- Gestational diabetes (diabetes in pregnancy).
- High blood pressure during pregnancy
- Pre-eclampsia
- Liver and gallbladder disorders during pregnancy
- Delivery complications
- Increased likelihood of induction of labor
- Slow progression of labor
- More likely to require a caesarean section
- Higher risk of cerebral palsy due to complicated birth
- Birth defects in the infant
- Higher body fat levels in the infant
- Poor IVF success and increased risk of premature birth
- Increased risk of obesity, diabetes and heart disease in the infant when they reach adulthood[66]

Most people just don't realize how dangerous it is to be obese while pregnant. The fetus is at significantly increased risk of the following birth defects:

- Spina bifida
- Exomphalos (a condition where the baby is born with its bowels and liver outside of the abdominal cavity)
- Orofacial clefts
- Congenital heart defects.
- Obese women are at increased risk of having a baby with neural tube defects. This increased risk is not completely abolished with folic acid supplements. Women with a BMI greater than or equal to 30 have a 15 percent increased

risk of having a child with a congenital heart defect. The more overweight a pregnant woman is, the greater the risk of heart defects in the infant, including atrial septal defects, hypoplastic left heart syndrome, aortic stenosis, pulmonic stenosis, and tetralogy of Fallot.[67, 68]

For every BMI unit above 25, there is a seven percent greater risk of abnormalities in the fetus. [69]

Diabetes

Overweight women and women with insulin resistance are at increased risk of developing diabetes in pregnancy, called gestational diabetes. During the second trimester of pregnancy, when the fetus is growing rapidly, hormones from the placenta start to reduce the ability of the mother's insulin to bind with insulin receptors in her body. Because the mother is less able to shuttle glucose out of her bloodstream, this guarantees a good supply of glucose for the fetus, which it needs for its development. To compensate for this situation, pregnant women's bodies produce between 1.5 and 2.5 times more insulin. Some pregnant women are unable to step up insulin production, therefore their blood sugar rises too high and they develop gestational diabetes. This happens in approximately seven to eight percent of all pregnancies.

Some women were already insulin resistant before they became pregnant. Their insulin receptors were already less sensitive to insulin than they should be, therefore the added stress of pregnancy leaves them unable to control their blood sugar and they too develop gestational diabetes. Women with polycystic ovarian syndrome and women with abdominal obesity are particularly prone to gestational diabetes. Tissue sensitivity to insulin is reduced by 50 to 60 percent by the third trimester of pregnancy.[70] Healthy women can cope with this, but overweight women, mineral deficient women and most women with a history of polycystic ovarian syndrome cannot cope. Their blood sugar rises too high, placing the health of their fetus at risk.

Gestational diabetes carries all the risks associated with obesity during pregnancy and more. Exposure to higher than normal levels of blood sugar makes the fetus grow bigger than normal.

It also forces the fetus' pancreas to secrete greater quantities of insulin in order to control its own blood sugar level. This can predispose the infant to blood sugar problems later in life. Pregnant women undergo routine blood tests to check their blood sugar level. Recent research has shown that a blood sugar level that is higher than ideal, but not high enough to be considered diabetes still has toxic effects on the fetus and increases the risk of adverse pregnancy outcomes. An ideal blood sugar level is less than 99 mg/dL (5.5 mmol/L).

High blood sugar causes most harm in the early stages of pregnancy, especially before the seventh week of gestation. Therefore all diabetic women wishing to become pregnant need to make sure their diabetes is well controlled, and their blood sugar level is as close as possible to normal. Several researchers believe that maternal diabetes and maternal obesity are leading factors responsible for the worldwide increase in congenital abnormalities. All overweight people have higher than ideal levels of inflammation in their bodies. This is mainly because fat cells produce a whole host of inflammatory chemicals that cause wear and tear in the body. High blood glucose and high blood insulin also promote inflammation.

Alcohol

Women who drink alcohol usually take longer to conceive than women who don't. Even women who drink five or less drinks a week take longer to conceive than women who don't drink weekly.[71] Alcohol reduces the production of progesterone, can inhibit ovulation and interferes with the transport of sperm through the fallopian tubes. Women who consume large amounts of alcohol, or drink frequently are more likely to suffer with menstrual disorders including painful periods, loss of menstrual periods or irregular menstruation. Alcohol worsens estrogen dominance and progesterone deficiency. It reduces the ability of the liver to break down estrogen.

In men, alcohol consumption leads to reduced semen volume, lower sperm count, reduced sperm motility and increased numbers of sperm with abnormal morphology. These effects are seen from research where men consumed 180mL of alcohol per day (brandy and whisky in this case) for a minimum of five days per week for at least a year.[72] In men alcohol promotes the conversion of testosterone to estrogen. This leads to lower blood testosterone levels and promotes weight gain and enlargement of the prostate gland.

Regular alcohol consumption also depletes the body of several vital nutrients. Nutrient deficiencies further aggravate infertility and increase the risk of adverse pregnancy outcomes. Alcohol can make you deficient in some nutrients because your body uses them up faster in order to break down the alcohol, or because you don't absorb nutrients as well (alcohol irritates the gastrointestinal lining and promotes an overgrowth of bad bowel bugs), or because alcohol causes you to lose more nutrients through your urine.

The following nutrients are depleted by alcohol. If you drink regularly or drink alcohol in large quantities, you should supplement with these nutrients before attempting conception:

All B vitamins, including folic acid (vitamin B9). B vitamins are essential for the development of the fetus' nervous system and for reducing the risk of neural tube defects, including spina bifida. Deficiency of these vitamins at the earliest stage of pregnancy (before many women realize they are pregnant) can already have adverse effects.

Magnesium

Zinc

Couples who are trying to conceive should avoid all alcohol, or limit intake to one or two drinks a week.

Caffeine

Caffeine doesn't affect every woman's ability to conceive, but some research has shown that women who consume more than 300mg of caffeine per day are twice as likely to experience infertility for a year or more.[73] Women who drink more than three cups of coffee in the first trimester of pregnancy have an increased risk of miscarriage. Caffeine consumption during pregnancy increases the risk of premature delivery, reduced fetal growth, and withdrawal symptoms in the baby after delivery.[74] Men who consume more than 700mg of caffeine per day have partners who take longer to conceive.[75] A study has shown that men who consumed more than 308mg of caffeine per day have 20 percent more DNA damage in their sperm than men who don't consume caffeine.[76]

See the table below for the caffeine content of foods and beverages:

Food	Caffeine content
Percolated coffee	60-120 mg / 250mL cup
Formulated caffeinated beverages or ' Energy' Drinks	80 mg / 250 mL can
Instant coffee (1 teaspoon/ cup)	60-80 mg / 250 mL cup
Tea	10-50 mg / 250 mL cup
Coca Cola	48.75mg / 375mL can
Milk Chocolate	20 mg / 100g bar

Source: Food Standards Australia

Cigarettes

The harmful effects of smoking are not limited to your lungs and respiratory tract. Smoking has a devastating effect on your reproductive tract. Female smokers are at increased risk of infertility, and even women exposed to second hand smoke experience difficulties conceiving. A study of 4,800 non-smoking women showed that those exposed to second hand smoke for six or more hours per day as children and adults had a 68 percent higher chance of infertility lasting more than one year, and suffered one or more miscarriages.[77]

Smoking while pregnant also increases the risk of placental problems, premature delivery and low birth weight. Cigarettes contain a plethora of toxic chemicals, including the heavy metal cadmium, which can interfere with ovulation. Women who smoke usually reach menopause sooner than non-smokers. Moderate smoking ages a woman's eggs by approximately ten years. This is extremely significant when you consider that a 25 year old smoker has the ovaries of a 35 year old.

Exposure to second hand smoke during pregnancy causes damage to the DNA inside a baby's cells. Research conducted at the University of Pittsburgh Graduate School of Public Health showed that newborns of non-smoking mums exposed to second hand smoke have genetic abnormalities (mutations) that are indistinguishable from those found in newborns of mothers who are smokers. Therefore, smoking while you are pregnant, or being exposed to cigarette smoke at that time, causes genetic damage to your baby. Therefore your infant may be born with faulty genes that can show up as birth defects, or affect their susceptibility to serious diseases like cancer.[78]

Medical research has been intensely focused on genes in recent years. Researchers have discovered the genes for breast cancer, Alzheimer's disease, depression, diabetes, the list goes on. All of these diseases are far more prevalent today than they were 50 years ago. Have you ever thought why these faulty genes are so prevalent today, whereas they were not around a short time ago? What causes these faulty genes? The answer is environmental factors, combined with nutrient deficiencies. Exposure to radiation and environmental chemicals at a critical time in life causes mutations to genes that then predispose individuals to a range of health problems. You are never more susceptible to harm caused by environmental agents than when you were inside your mother's uterus. Therefore everything a pregnant woman comes in contact with has a potentially harmful effect on her baby. Early childhood is also a vulnerable time when the DNA inside the cells of the body is very vulnerable to environmental harm.

Women who smoke are more likely to have children who go on to become infertile. A study published in The Journal of Clinical Investigation showed that smoking before, during and even after pregnancy puts baby girls at greater risk of infertility. Earlier research found the same outcome in baby boys. This is not surprising, considering that a woman's ovaries contain all the eggs she will ever have while she is still inside her mother's uterus. The ovaries are fully formed, with all eggs inside before a woman is born. In men, the testes contain the precursor cells that will become sperm before a man is born. Smoking before and during pregnancy limits the reproductive potential of your children.

In men, cigarette smoking reduces sperm count and sperm motility.[79] The semen of male smokers is higher in free radicals and the DNA inside the sperm is more likely to be damaged. The sperm of men who smoke have a reduced ability to penetrate and fertilize an egg.[80]

Harmful fats

The type of fat you consume affects your ability to become pregnant. All natural fats are beneficial; saturated, monounsaturated and polyunsaturated fats are all beneficial to your health if they are in their natural form. There is a very strong link between trans fatty acids and infertility. These are man made fats that have had their structure changed. Vegetable oils are naturally shaped in a "cis" form, but when they are partially hydrogenated, the fats change into a "trans" form. Trans fatty acids are found widely in processed and packaged foods that contain vegetable oil or have been fried in vegetable oil. You can find reference to trans fatty acids on the nutrition information panel of packaged foods, or the term vegetable oil in an ingredients list means the product probably contains trans fats.

Trans fats can prevent ovulation. Researchers at the Harvard School of Public Health in the USA have discovered that the more trans fats a woman eats, the more likely she is to be infertile. Dr Jorge Chavarro and his team found that consuming just four grams of trans fats per day can significantly increase a woman's risk of infertility. This is a tiny amount that is extremely easy to consume if you regularly eat takeaway food, biscuits, cake, crackers, potato or corn chips, pretzels and similar foods. Trans fats extend the shelf life of processed foods, so they are popular with the food industry. In recent years the quantity of trans fats in foods has fallen dramatically because of negative publicity they have received, but they are still present in many foods and it is easy to consume a mere four grams a day.

The researchers at Harvard analyzed data from 18,555 healthy American women who participated in the Nurses' Health Study. All of the women were trying to get pregnant between 1991 and 1999. The results showed that for every two percent increase in calories a woman received from trans fats instead of omega 6 polyunsaturated fats, the risk of infertility jumped by 79 percent.[81]

The researchers believe that trans fats interfere with a woman's ability to ovulate because they interfere with insulin sensitivity and glucose metabolism and promote inflammation. Women who do fall pregnant and consume trans fats place their baby at risk. Trans fats cross the placenta, become incorporated into the baby's cells and increase the risk of low birth weight. Pregnant women who consume trans fats are at increased risk of high blood pressure and pre-eclampsia.

Fat is very beneficial to your health and fertility but you must consume fat in its natural form. Oily fish, avocados, raw nuts and seeds, coconut milk and extra virgin olive oil are all extremely beneficial natural forms of fat. Try to include these foods in your diet regularly.

Genetically modified foods

Genetically modified foods are bad news for several reasons, and now animal studies have shown they can cause infertility. Research conducted in Austria showed that genetically modified corn has a harmful effect on the reproductive system. Very few long term studies have been carried out on genetically modified foods. This research was requested by the Austrian Health Ministry and studied the effects of genetically modified (GM) corn on mice. Over a period of 20 weeks it became apparent that the fertility of mice fed genetically modified corn was seriously impaired, with fewer offspring than mice fed conventional corn. When several generations of mice were studied, the GM corn fed mice produced significantly fewer offspring, particularly in the third and fourth generations. The offspring were also of lower birth weight. The mice eating conventional corn reproduced more rapidly.[82]

The introduction of genetically modified food is an experiment we will learn the results of in the coming years. The following genetically modified foods have been approved by sale in Australia and the USA:

GM corn

GM cotton. Cottonseed oil is used widely in processed foods and often labeled simply as vegetable oil.

GM soybeans

GM potatoes

GM canola

These items can only be consumed in processed foods at this

stage; they are not currently sold as fresh foods. Genetically modified foods must be identified on food labels but there are exceptions. If the GM food makes up less than one percent of the ingredients list, it does not have to be stated on the label. Also if the GM food is a component of vegetable oil, it does not have to appear on the label. Genetically modified foods are most likely to be present in highly processed foods, such as cheap chocolate bars with more than half a dozen ingredients. If you eat basic, simple, fresh and unprocessed foods, you will be unlikely to consume genetically modified foods. Unfortunately many takeaway food outlets use cottonseed oil or canola oil for frying, and this is likely to be genetically modified.

Exercise

Too much exercise or too little exercise can negatively impact fertility. Too little exercise is the much more common scenario of course. Lack of exercise increases the risk of becoming overweight, and overweight women are more likely to have anovulatory menstrual cycles. That is, they are more likely to have menstrual periods in which no ovulation occurs. Overweight women are also more prone to developing polycystic ovarian syndrome (PCOS). Women with PCOS have insulin resistance (syndrome X) and it is their high blood insulin level that interferes with ovulation and progesterone production. Regular exercise helps to keep blood insulin levels down and body fat levels within a healthy range. Regular exercise, combined with a low carbohydrate eating plan is one of the fastest and easiest ways to enable an infertile woman with PCOS to achieve pregnancy.

Exercise needs to be continued during pregnancy, but at a lower intensity. Exercising during pregnancy reduces the risk of high blood pressure, gestational diabetes and giving birth to an abnormally large baby. Some research has shown it may make labor less painful. A small study conducted in Brazil found that women who exercised while pregnant had a reduced need for anesthesia while giving birth. 71 pregnant women were studied; 34 of them performed water aerobics three times a week for 50 minutes each, and the remaining 37 women did not exercise. All of the 71 women were matched for age, weight, education and previous births. All of the women were healthy and there was no difference among them in the length of their labor, type of delivery or health of their newborn. However, the study showed that only 27 percent of the exercisers requested pain medication during labor, compared with 65 percent of the non-exercisers.[83]

Too much exercise can cause menstrual disturbances and infertility, but this is mainly seen in athletes and under weight women. Vigorous exercise is capable of inhibiting ovulation. A study conducted in Norway found that exercising to exhaustion increased the risk of infertility by 2.3 times. Those findings were independent of age, smoking or body mass index.[84]

The risk is increased much further for under weight women. The loss of menstrual periods is called amenorrhea, and this occurs in between one and 44 percent of female athletes. Inadequate progesterone production is thought to affect up to 79 percent of all female athletes intermittently. This includes recreational runners who have regular menstrual periods.[85]

Problems with progesterone production are commonly referred to as luteal phase defects. The corpus luteum left behind after ovulation cannot produce sufficient progesterone and this usually produces a short luteal phase (less than ten days). Therefore the second half of the menstrual cycle is shorter than normal and this can cause symptoms such as premenstrual syndrome, abnormal uterine bleeding, infertility and miscarriage.

Lack of exercise and obesity in men is associated with lower sperm counts and high numbers of abnormal sperm. However, extreme exercise can also impact male fertility. Exercising to the point of exhaustion, particularly in long distance runners, triathletes and cyclists is associated with poor semen parameters. Exhaustive exercise increases free radical damage and oxidative stress in the body; this increases the amount of DNA damage inside sperm. Moderate exercise has a beneficial effect because it increases the activity of antioxidant enzymes in the body.

Cycling is potentially the most harmful type of exercise to male fertility because sitting on a conventional bicycle saddle can cause compression and damage to the pudendal nerves and arteries that travel to the penis. This increases the risk of erectile dysfunction. Alternative bicycle seats are available that are shaped differently and distribute body weight on the sit bones of the backside.

Stress

Stress is not good for fertility, but you have probably heard that several times already! Stress is the factor most likely to disrupt a woman's menstrual cycle. Stress suppresses the brain's production of hormones that control the ovaries and stimulate the development of eggs. Stress also increases the production of the hormone prolactin; this can suppress ovulation, can cause PMS and may lead to a temporary loss of menstrual periods (amenorrhea). Prolonged stress also leads to an elevation of the adrenal hormone cortisol. Cortisol and progesterone are both steroid hormones manufactured out of cholesterol; highly stressed women experience a reduction in progesterone levels because their body is busy manufacturing cortisol. Your body perceives stress as a threat to your survival; therefore it wisely shuts down your reproductive system, fearing that it may not be safe to procreate at this time. In men, social and psychological stress can result in lowered testosterone and decreased sperm production.[86]

Pharmaceutical drugs

Some commonly used medication can increase the risk of infertility. Non-steroidal anti-inflammatory drugs such as aspirin, ibuprofen, Voltarin (diclofenac), Ponstan (mefenamic acid) and Aleve and Naprogesic (naproxen) can prevent ovulation or cause premature rupture of the ovarian follicle. This is also the case for the anti-inflammatory drugs Celebrex (celecoxib) and Vioxx (rofecoxib) These drugs also increase the risk of miscarriage if used during pregnancy.

Nutrient deficiencies

A simple vitamin or mineral deficiency can be responsible for infertility. It is vitally important to correct any nutritional deficiencies before conception occurs. Ideally you need to clean up your diet and supplement with the right nutrients for at least three months before you attempt to conceive. This will ensure your body is the best possible environment for a growing baby. You want your eggs and your partner's sperm to be as healthy as possible, as they are the foundation of your child's health. The healthier you are before and during pregnancy, the healthier your child will be also.

Multivitamin use during pregnancy significantly reduces the risk of cancer in your children

Research carried out at the Toronto Hospital for Sick Children found that babies of mothers who took multivitamins throughout pregnancy were far less likely to develop cancer. These babies had:

47 percent less neuroblastoma. This is the most common type of cancer in infancy and develops from nerve tissue.

39 percent less leukemia

27 percent less brain tumors[87]

It's amazing to think what a profound effect a simple multivitamin had, since most multivitamins actually contain tiny and suboptimal quantities of each vitamin and mineral.

Most people are nutrient deficient

Clearly, being nutrient deficient increases the risk of adverse outcomes for you and your baby. Nutrient deficiencies are frighteningly common. Very few people have a perfect diet; and even if your diet is perfectly healthy, food sold today is far lower in nutrients than food sold a hundred years ago. Over farming has depleted the soil of minerals, and most fruit and vegetables sold today were picked many months before they are eventually sold. They have been kept in cold storage or even frozen. Vitamins are more delicate than minerals and handling food this way quickly depletes fresh produce of vitamins.

Ideally you should try to eat organic fruit and vegetables. Clearly this is often not possible, due to lack of availability, cost and low quality. If you can grow some of your own fruit, vegetables and herbs, that is ideal. Also try to shop in local farmers markets, as the produce is usually locally grown and much fresher. Every single vitamin and mineral has an important role to play in helping you to conceive and maintain a healthy pregnancy; however we will now look at the nutrients you are most likely to be deficient in, as well as the most important nutrients for fertility.

By optimizing your health and nutrient intake before you fall pregnant, you can greatly reduce the risk of congenital abnormalities, miscarriage, insufficient fetal growth, premature birth and pre-eclampsia.[88] Being nutrient deficient in the first trimester of pregnancy increases the risk of obesity, heart disease and high cholesterol in your child in adulthood. Your diet at the time you conceive sets the course for your child's future health. Half of your child's DNA will come from you, and the other half comes from your partner. Apart from an occasional mutation, deletion or duplication of information, the DNA is supposed to remain unchanged between generations. Exposure to radiation and environmental chemicals, particularly when combined with nutrient deficiencies can cause actual damage to genes. But it is far more likely that the genes you pass on will remain the same, but they could function differently.

The environment you are exposed to, whether or not you smoke, how stressed you are, and the toxins you come into contact with on a daily basis can change how your genes are expressed and how they function. Those changes can be passed down to your offspring, even if the actual DNA sequence itself does not change. These changes are referred to as epigenetic changes and they occur via a process known as DNA methylation. This is basically where molecules bind to our DNA and either turn on or turn off genes. B vitamins are extremely essential for healthy methylation. Deficiency of B vitamins makes your genes more susceptible to harm caused by environmental chemicals and toxins. Folic acid, vitamin B12, B6, vitamin D as well as selenium are the most important nutrients to protect your DNA. If your DNA has undergone harmful epigenetic changes, you will pass those on to your children, who will pass them onto their children, and the health of future generations will deteriorate. You can reduce the risk of this scenario by paying close attention to your diet before and during pregnancy. You have an enormous amount of influence over your genes.

Nutrient deficiencies caused by the oral contraceptive pill

The pill causes several nutrient deficiencies in the body, particularly:

- Magnesium
- Zinc
- Folic acid
- B vitamins - particularly B6, B5 and B2
- Vitamin C
- Vitamin A
- Selenium

Each of these nutrients is critical for fertility, a healthy pregnancy and a healthy baby. You have probably not taken the pill for at least a year, but unless you have been taking these nutrients in supplement form, your body is probably still lacking them.

We will now look at the key individual nutrients required for fertility:

Folic acid/folate

Folic acid is also known as vitamin B9. It is certainly the most well publicized nutrient required for a healthy pregnancy. Folic acid is required in the earliest stages of pregnancy; therefore it is ideal to take a supplement for three months before you try to conceive. Folic acid is a water soluble nutrient, therefore does not remain in your body for long. This means it is vital to receive plenty of this nutrient each day. Folic acid helps to reduce the risk of neural tube defects such as spina bifida and cleft palate in the infant, but it also helps to reduce the risk of congenital heart defects and childhood cancer. Neural tube defects are one of the most common birth defects and occur in approximately one in 1000 infants in Western nations. In the third to fourth week of pregnancy, specialized cells of the fetus begin to fuse and form the neural tube. When the neural tube does not close properly, a neural tube defect occurs. It is basically an opening in the spinal cord or brain.

Taking a folic acid supplement greatly reduces the risk of neural tube defects, but it does not eliminate the risk completely.

Maternal obesity, maternal diabetes and cigarette smoking are all associated with an increased risk. Research has shown that taking a folic acid supplement for at least a year before becoming pregnant cuts the risk of having a premature baby in half.[89] Folic acid is found in foliage; therefore green leafy vegetables are an excellent source of this nutrient. Eating plenty of raw vegetables is vitally important, but a folic acid supplement will guarantee that you are receiving enough of this nutrient. We recommend you take 500 micrograms of folic acid per day with food.

Selenium

Selenium is vitally important for healthy thyroid gland function and a healthy immune system. All women with a thyroid condition need extra selenium. All women and men with autoimmune disease, allergies and excess inflammation need more selenium. This mineral is excellent for reducing thyroid antibodies, sperm antibodies and other auto-antibodies. Selenium helps to protect the DNA inside your cells from damage; deficiency increases the risk of miscarriage and the risk of genetic abnormalities and congenital disorders in offspring.

Selenium also helps your body to fight viral infections. It is essential to have optimum selenium levels in your body while you are pregnant, as this will help to protect you against colds and flu at this time. Pregnant women are at greater risk of serious infections. Selenium is extremely important for male fertility and helps to reduce the numbers of abnormal sperm. Selenium protects the DNA inside sperm from damage, therefore reduces the risk of a male passing on genetic defects to his children. It is impossible to obtain optimum levels of selenium through diet because most soils around the world are selenium deficient. A nutritional supplement is the only way to guarantee you are receiving adequate selenium to enhance fertility and protect your child. We recommend you take 200 micrograms of selenium per day.

Iodine

Iodine is critically important for the health of your thyroid gland. Thyroid hormones are made of a combination of iodine and the amino acid tyrosine. Iodine deficiency is incredibly common and this partly explains the high rate of thyroid disorders in the world. Sub-optimum thyroid function is a common cause of infertility. Iodine deficiency also increases the risk of ovarian cysts.

Iodine deficiency in pregnant women is an extremely common problem and can have disastrous consequences. When you are pregnant, your thyroid gland needs to pump out much higher amounts of hormones, in order to provide for your baby before its thyroid gland has developed. If you don't have enough iodine in your diet, your thyroid gland will not be able to do this. Iodine deficiency during pregnancy increases the risk of gestational high blood pressure, miscarriage and stillbirth.[90]

The main role of thyroid hormone in the fetus is nervous system development. Therefore iodine deficiency at this time greatly increases the risk of brain damage, learning difficulties, lowered IQ and hearing loss in the fetus. Australian research has shown that approximately half of the pregnant women in NSW, Victoria and Tasmania are iodine deficient.[91] What a terrifying concept! Iodine also has a natural antiseptic effect in your body and helps to protect you against infections. This is particularly important during pregnancy.

It is very difficult to obtain enough iodine through diet alone. Most of the world's iodine is found in the oceans. Therefore seafood is traditionally the richest source of iodine, however much of the fish available for sale now has been farmed, and therefore is a poor source of iodine. Seaweed is very rich in iodine, but it is not commonly consumed in large enough quantities. Iodized salt provides some iodine, but it is important to avoid salt that contains a free flow agent because that is aluminum; added to prevent the salt from clumping. Sea salt barely contains any iodine. If you consume raw cabbage, broccoli, cauliflower or Brussels sprouts, you will need extra iodine because these vegetables contain goitrogens, which reduce the ability of your thyroid gland to absorb iodine. Cooking those vegetables largely inactivates goitrogens. Selenium deficiency exacerbates the effects of iodine deficiency.

The Recommended Daily Intake of iodine is 150 micrograms per day. This figure leaps up to 220 micrograms for pregnant women and 290 micrograms for breast feeding women. Very few women are able to achieve that level of intake without a supplement. You can check your body's level of iodine through a urine test. See chapter 10 for details.

Zinc

Zinc deficiency is one of the most common mineral deficiencies among women, especially vegetarian women and women who have taken the oral contraceptive pill. Furthermore, taking an iron supplement reduces the ability of your body to absorb zinc, therefore may compound the problem. Zinc is vitally important for healthy immune system function and deficiency can result in low levels of white blood cells. Zinc is particularly important for women with immune system disorders that are contributing to infertility. Gluten intolerant men and women are at increased risk of zinc deficiency.

Being zinc deficient while pregnant places you at heightened risk of contracting an infection, and once your baby is born, it too is at increased risk of infections. Zinc deficiency increases the risk of pregnancy complications; specifically premature labor, low birth weight, delivery difficulties and congenital abnormalities in the baby.[92] Zinc is one of the most important nutrients for male fertility, and is required for testosterone production and healthy sperm production. Zinc supplementation can increase the quantity and quality of sperm.

Good food sources of zinc include oysters (don't eat them raw), red meat, poultry and nuts. Grains can reduce zinc absorption; that's another reason to keep their consumption to a minimum. Correcting a zinc deficiency with food alone is a very slow process, therefore a zinc supplement is recommended. You can take between 20 and 40 mg of zinc per day in supplement form.

Vitamin B12

Vitamin B12 is required for the activation of folic acid. You will not get maximum benefits from a folic acid supplement unless you have optimum levels of vitamin B12 in your body. Vitamin B12 helps to protect the DNA inside the eggs and sperm from harm, therefore reduces the risk of the parents passing genetic defects on to the fetus. It is also required for correct cell division and nervous system development in the fetus. Vegetarians and people with digestive problems resulting in poor absorption are very prone to B12 deficiency. This vitamin is only present in animal products, such as meat, poultry and fish. We recommend a supplement of 500 micrograms before conception and during pregnancy. Your vitamin B12 level can be measured in a blood test.

Vitamin C

Vitamin C is a powerful antioxidant and helps to protect the eggs and sperm from free radical damage. Vitamin C can help progesterone deficient women to become pregnant. Inadequate progesterone production in the second half of the menstrual cycle is commonly referred to as luteal phase defect. In a study of infertile women with luteal phase defect, supplementing with 750mg of vitamin C per day for six months resulted in a pregnancy rate of 25 percent, compared to 11 percent in the women not taking a supplement.[93] Vitamin C is crucial for the structural integrity of the uterus and helps to reduce the risk of uterine rupture during pregnancy and labor. You can take between 2 and 5 grams of vitamin C per day in supplement form. Don't take it all in one go; spread your intake throughout the day.

Vitamin E

Vitamin E is a powerful antioxidant that helps to protect cell membranes from free radical damage. In this way it helps to improve the health of eggs and sperm. Vitamin E deficiency in animals is a well known cause of infertility. In humans, research has shown that women given 200 IU per day and men given 100 IU per day of vitamin E showed a significant increase in fertility.[94]

Iron

You are probably well aware that iron requirements increase during pregnancy, but you need ample iron in your body in order to become pregnant. Iron deficiency increases the risk of anovulation; meaning iron deficiency can prevent you from ovulating. If you do manage to conceive while iron deficient, you are at greater risk of miscarriage. Iron deficiency is quite common in women; particularly women with heavy menstrual periods and women who don't eat much red meat. Iron deficiency causes anemia; symptoms of anemia include:

- Fatigue
- Dizziness
- Low blood pressure
- Breathlessness and low exercise tolerance
- Low body temperature and being sensitive to the cold. Sometimes this is mistaken for an under active thyroid gland.
- Headaches
- Weak and brittle nails
- Tinnitus (ringing in the ears)

You should only take an iron supplement if a blood test has shown you to be iron deficient. See chapter 10 for information on blood tests. Good food sources of iron include red meat, fish, egg yolks, poultry, apricots and green leafy vegetables.

Vitamin D

Vitamin D deficiency is extremely wide spread and can greatly impact fertility. Vitamin D deficiency can inhibit ovulation, and women with polycystic ovarian syndrome are particularly likely to be vitamin D deficient. A study conducted at Yale University School of Medicine found that 93 percent of infertile women were vitamin D deficient!

According to Dr Lubna Pal, from Yale, "Of note, not a single patient with either ovulatory disturbance or polycystic ovary syndrome demonstrated normal Vitamin D levels; 39 per cent of those with ovulatory disturbance and 38 per cent of those with PCOS had serum 25OH D levels consistent with deficiency. Given the pandemic of Vitamin D insufficiency, if indeed our observations are substantiated, aggressive repletion with Vitamin D may emerge as an alternative approach to facilitate ovulation resumption with minimal to no risk for ovarian hyperstimulation syndrome or multiple pregnancy."[95] To be classed as vitamin D deficient, you really need to have extremely low blood levels of this nutrient. Far more women have suboptimal vitamin D levels, which still greatly impairs their fertility and overall health.

Vitamin D deficiency increases the risk of immune mediated infertility because deficiency is associated with high levels of inflammation and allergies. Women with optimum blood vitamin D levels have far more success with IVF. They experience significantly increased implantation rates and rates of clinical pregnancy.[96]

Vitamin D deficiency increases the risk of pre-eclampsia and increases the risk of birth complications that make a caesarean section necessary. Taking a vitamin D supplement for three months before conception and throughout pregnancy is essential unless you spend most of your time outdoors. You will need to have your blood vitamin D level monitored to make sure it remains between 40 and 60 ng/mL (100 and 150 nmol/L).

Breast milk is a notoriously poor source of vitamin D and this can have terrible health consequences for infants. Most women are so vitamin D deficient that their bodies do not have enough to spare to secrete into breast milk. Vitamin D deficiency in infancy places a child at substantially increased risk of all autoimmune diseases, including type 1 diabetes and multiple sclerosis. Deficiency also increases the risk of rickets, asthma and eczema in infants. Babies born with vitamin D deficiency are twice as likely to develop schizophrenia later in life. According to Dr Michael Holick, a world authority on vitamin D, lactating women who do not receive regular midday sun exposure should be taking 6000 IU of vitamin D per day in capsule form. This is a general recommendation, and some individuals will require more or less; that is why it is important to have regular vitamin D blood tests.

Magnesium

Magnesium is important while trying to conceive for several reasons. Magnesium helps insulin to work more efficiently in your body, therefore all overweight women, women with insulin resistance (syndrome X), diabetes and women with polycystic ovarian syndrome greatly benefit from magnesium. Most Australians do not receive enough magnesium through their diet. Magnesium is found in green vegetables, brown rice, nuts and several other foods but it is difficult to obtain enough through food. When you are stressed, your body uses up far greater quantities of magnesium, and alcohol increases magnesium excretion.

You need plenty of magnesium in your body in order to utilize vitamin D properly, as all of the enzymes that metabolize vitamin D require magnesium. Magnesium is also required for correct DNA replication; therefore it helps to reduce the risk of genetic damage in your offspring. Magnesium deficiency significantly increases the risk of pre-eclampsia. Magnesium has a relaxing effect on the nerves and muscles of your body and should help you to feel significantly less stressed. This is very valuable while trying to conceive. A magnesium supplement should be taken for at least three months before attempting conception, and right throughout pregnancy and lactation. An ideal dose is 400 mg daily.

The fertility diet: how to get pregnant fast

The following diet and lifestyle guidelines will help to provide your body with the nutrients it needs most, reduce the level of inflammation inside your body and calm down an over active immune system. Everybody's health would benefit from following these guidelines and they help to reduce your risk of chronic diseases, including cancer and heart disease. However, in the short term, these guidelines will improve your chances of conceiving and maintaining a healthy pregnancy to full term. They will also help to improve your child's immune system and reduce the risk of allergies and immune dysfunction in your child.

Pregnancy is a major stress on a woman's body. Your body is wise; it will not allow you to become pregnant if a pregnancy would be a threat to your health. The average person's diet is nutrient deficient. Even people who think they have a healthy diet typically suffer with several nutrient deficiencies. These will often not be apparent. Typically they will not produce any symptoms, so you will not be aware of their existence. However, with the stress of pregnancy on your body, nutrient deficiencies can have serious consequences.

Rates of pregnancy complications, delivery complications and maternal death during delivery are very high among women in third world countries. This is largely because of the severe nutrient deficiencies these women suffer. Well, American women have been shown to be very deficient in key nutrients such as iodine, vitamin D, omega 3 fats, magnesium, zinc, selenium and others. Even a well fed population can be very undernourished. These diet guidelines will reduce inflammation, improve your immune system and provide the nutrients your body needs to achieve conception and a healthy pregnancy. Excess inflammation is behind several causes of infertility and pregnancy complications, and these diet guidelines address that.

Foods to include in your diet

Increase your intake of vegetables

You need to consume at least seven serves of vegetables each day and some of them need to be raw. A serve is roughly half a cup of chopped vegetables. Vegetables are high in fiber, vitamins, minerals and antioxidants. The fiber in vegetables will help to keep your bowel movements regular. Most people eat at least three times a day; therefore you should be having between one and three bowel movements each day. The fiber in vegetables is mostly soluble fiber and acts as food for good bacteria in your digestive tract. The fiber that encourages the growth of beneficial bacteria is called a prebiotic, whereas the good bugs themselves are called a probiotic.

Vegetables are high in vitamins and minerals, and most of them are very low in sugar, with the exception of potato, sweet potato and parsnip. Most vegetables are far lower in sugar than fruit; therefore you need to eat a lot more vegetables than fruit. Please limit your fruit intake to two pieces per day. It is especially important for overweight men and women and women with polycystic ovarian syndrome to limit their fruit intake.

Along with vitamins and minerals, vegetables and fruit are both high in phyto-chemicals. These are plant compounds that give fruit and vegetables their color, and they act as antioxidants. The antioxidants in fruit and vegetables are strongly anti-inflammatory. Please eat a wide variety of vegetables each day and make sure you eat different colored vegetables.

Consume adequate protein

Your body is largely made of protein and you need to consume enough protein in your diet for tissue repair, muscle function, hormone and enzyme production, immune system function and several other reasons. Animal foods are the richest source of protein; these include fish, poultry, eggs, red meat and dairy products. We recommend you avoid dairy products, and will explain why further along in this chapter. All processed red meat needs to be avoided; this means deli meat, ham, sausages (organic, preservative free are fine), bacon, corned meat, salami and other preserved meat. Please consume fish, poultry and eggs more often than you consume red meat. If you can obtain and afford organic animal protein, it is preferable. Pasture fed (grass fed) meat is better than grain fed meat. The seafood you consume needs to be wild, not farmed. Farmed seafood is not fed its natural diet and is low in omega 3 fat and iodine. It also contains residues of antibiotics, dyes and other chemicals. Unfortunately most fresh salmon is farmed. Some canned salmon is wild.

Protein is also found in nuts, seeds, legumes and grains, but in smaller quantities and the protein in these foods is said to be incomplete because none of these foods alone contains all eight essential amino acids. Vegetarians can combine these foods in their diet in order to obtain sufficient protein. Protein powder is also a valuable source of protein. We recommend you avoid soy protein powder; whey protein powder is okay unless you are very sensitive to dairy products. You can also obtain protein powder made from yellow peas or rice; this is easy to digest and unlikely to cause allergies.

You need to consume protein at each meal; this will help to keep your blood sugar stable and greatly reduce hunger and cravings. Increasing your protein intake is an excellent way to lose weight because it will keep you full for longer and reduce sugar and carbohydrate cravings. A higher protein, low carbohydrate diet is essential for the treatment of polycystic ovarian syndrome and obesity. We have two books that contain a low carbohydrate eating plan and recipes, they are: *Can't Lose Weight? Unlock the Secrets that* keep you fat and *Diabetes Type 2: You can Reverse it Naturally.* You don't have to be a diabetic to benefit from a low carbohydrate diet.

Eat plenty of good fats

You need to consume adequate amounts of the right fat because fat is a building block of sex hormones and some fats have anti-inflammatory actions. Humans need both omega 3 and omega 6 fatty acids; both of them are essential for our bodies. Omega 6 fats are easily obtained in the diet because they are found in so many foods; nuts, seeds and vegetable oil are all a good source of omega 6 fats. In fact most people consume far too much omega 6 fat in relation to omega 3 fat. This is easy to do because processed foods usually contain soy, corn, sunflower, canola, cottonseed or safflower oil, all of which are high in omega 6 fats.

Modern farming methods mean that livestock, poultry and eggs are high in omega 6 fats because the animals were raised on grains, rather than pasture fed. Pasture fed (grass fed) animals produce meat that is far higher in beneficial omega 3 fats. Consuming too much omega 6 fat is a problem because omega 6 fats are used as a building block to manufacture inflammatory chemicals in the body. Therefore a high intake of omega 6 relative to omega 3 fat promotes systemic inflammation and immune system dysfunction. This imbalance in fatty acids is thought to increase the risk of not only infertility, but also inflammation, cancer, depression and heart disease.

It is very difficult to obtain sufficient omega 3 fats in modern diets. The particularly beneficial omega 3 fats are called EPA and DHA and they are only found in seafood (and the algae that fish consume). Omega 3 fats have an anti-inflammatory effect because consuming them turns on genes that increase the production of anti-inflammatory chemicals in your body. Omega 3 fats also reduce inflammation by inhibiting the activation of a highly inflammatory molecule called NF-kB (when activated, this molecule triggers the release of a flood of inflammatory chemicals). The best dietary source of omega 3 fats is oily fish such as sardines, mackerel, anchovies, herrings and salmon. Please only consume wild fish, not farmed fish. For good health it is recommended you consume these fish three times a week. However, people who have a health problem (such as infertility or immune system disorders) need greater quantities of omega 3 fats that only a fish oil supplement can provide. An ideal dose of omega 3 fats is approximately 1.8 grams per day of EPA and 1.2 grams per day of DHA. It is usually easier to achieve these high doses with liquid fish oil.

Omega 3 fats are some of the most powerful anti-inflammatory substances in nature, and taking a fish oil supplement in the right dose is enormously beneficial for autoimmune and inflammatory conditions. Most of the inflammatory chemicals that are found in high levels in people with autoimmune disease are made out of omega 6 fats. Reducing your intake of these fats, while supplementing with omega 3 fats greatly suppresses the production of inflammatory chemicals (cytokines). Clinical trials have shown omega 3 fats to be of therapeutic benefit in just about all autoimmune disease.[97]

Vegetarian foods such as flaxseeds, walnuts, pecans and chia seeds contain the omega 3 fat called alpha linolenic acid (ALA). ALA is a precursor to EPA and DHA but your body converts only between five and 18 percent into these beneficial fats; the rest is used for energy or stored as body fat. Therefore these foods are not a reliable source of omega 3 fat. We recommend fish oil instead.

Monounsaturated fats in olive oil, avocados and macadamia nuts are also anti-inflammatory and you should include them in your diet regularly. Monounsaturated fats help to keep the blood thin and reduce the risk of blood clots. In addition to being high in good fats, olive oil contains powerful antioxidants that dampen down inflammation and benefit the immune system. Spanish research has found that extra virgin olive oil exerts a beneficial effect on 98 genes that regulate inflammation.[98] The polyphenol antioxidants in olives are called tyrosols and they are extremely effective at mopping up the inflammation generated by free radicals in the body. These antioxidants are not present in refined olive oil; therefore you must use cold pressed, extra virgin olive oil to obtain these benefits.

Eat lots of nuts and seeds

Nuts and seeds should form a regular part of your diet. They are high in beneficial fats, fiber, vitamins, minerals and antioxidants and are anti-inflammatory. Because nuts and seeds are high in good fats, they can become rancid easily. Therefore you should only purchase raw nuts (not roasted) and not salted. All salted nuts available for sale have been roasted. Heating nuts can damage the delicate fatty acids inside them, and if you purchase roasted nuts, they were roasted a long time ago. By the time you purchase and eat them, the fats are damaged and no longer beneficial.

Even though nuts and seeds are high in fat, you would have to eat a lot of them to become overweight. Numerous studies have shown that nut eaters are slimmer and less prone to diabetes and heart disease than people who don't eat nuts. Include some or all of the following nuts and seeds in your diet: almonds, hazelnuts, Brazil nuts, pecans, walnuts, pine nuts, pistachios, sunflower seeds, sesame seeds, pumpkin seeds, chia seeds and flaxseeds. Flaxseeds must be ground into a powder in a grinder or food processor in order to be digestible. If you have a nut allergy, or eating nuts makes you feel unwell, please avoid them.

Include herbs and spices in your diet

Herbs and spices are an excellent source of antioxidants and anti-inflammatory compounds. Try to include fresh herbs in your meals regularly. Examples include parsley, rocket, coriander, basil, oregano, marjoram, sorrel and mint. It is best to grow some herbs at home, either in a vegetable patch or in pots. Herbs take very little looking after and if you grow them yourself you know they will be organic and fresh. Leafy plants lose nutrients as soon as they are pulled from the ground, so you will be receiving substantially more nutrients if you grow some herbs yourself rather than purchasing them. Spices are also a valuable addition to your diet. Examples of beneficial spices include turmeric, cumin, paprika and coriander.

Include minimal quantities of gluten free grains and starches in your diet

We recommend you keep your intake of grains to a minimum for several reasons. Grains promote inflammation (particularly gluten containing grains); they increase acidity levels in the body and can impair the absorption of minerals. If you are overweight, have syndrome X (insulin resistance) or polycystic ovarian syndrome, it is vital you eliminate grains from your diet. This is because grains and starches increase insulin, and therefore can inhibit ovulation. Everyone else can eat small quantities of rice (preferably brown), potatoes, corn, amaranth and quinoa.

Consume plenty of healthy fluids

Purified water, herbal tea and green tea are all healthy fluids you should consume abundantly. Drinking plenty of fluids will increase your energy level, speed up your metabolism, cleanse your bowel and help with weight loss.

Healthy lifestyle habits

Exercise and good sleep are essential

People who exercise regularly are known to have lower levels of inflammatory markers in their bloodstream. Exercise particularly lowers a compound called C-reactive protein, which is manufactured in the liver. Fat cells, (particularly those over the abdomen) produce a host of inflammatory chemicals; therefore overweight people have higher levels of chronic inflammation. Exercise promotes a healthy body weight, therefore keeps inflammation in check via reduction in body fat. Sleep has a powerfully restorative effect on the immune system and nervous system. Try to get seven to eight hours of sleep each night. The quality of your sleep will probably improve once you follow our diet guidelines.

Manage stress

Chronic stress causes your adrenal glands to pump out sustained high levels of cortisol. Over time this will cause an imbalance in your immune system and make you more prone to allergies, autoimmune disease and cancer. You can be following a healthy diet, taking supplements and exercising regularly, but if stress is a major part of your life, you will not achieve optimum health. In the majority of cases, whether or not we become stressed by an event depends on the way we perceive it. The way you think and the way you speak to yourself in your mind determines how upset you become by events in your life.

A number of strategies are very helpful for managing stress, these include:

Exercise. Back when we were hunters and gatherers, living in caves, stress usually meant a physical threat; often that something wanted to catch you and eat you. Today, you can be sitting at your desk all day, stressed by deadlines and angry customers. This is a dramatic change that our bodies do not cope well with. When you are stressed, your body releases hormones that prepare you for movement; "fight or flight" hormones. Sustained high levels of these hormones causes inflammation in your body, high blood pressure, high blood sugar and makes you more prone to developing the diseases of Western society.

When you are stressed, your body wants to move. Therefore regular exercise is the best way to dissipate stress hormones, elevate your mood and improve your energy. Ideally you would exercise for 30 to 60 minutes most days of the week and it would be a form of exercise that raises your heart rate and makes you huff and puff. Gentle exercise like yoga, tai chi, stretching and pilates is also immensely beneficial. Regular exercisers cope better with stress than people who don't exercise.

Avoid stimulants and excess alcohol. Sugar, caffeine and cigarettes can all lift your mood, help you to concentrate and give you a burst of energy when you really need it. Unfortunately over the long term these substances rob your body of energy and nutrients and greatly increase the risk of many health problems. Conversely, alcohol can help you wind down at the end of a long and stressful day but daily consumption or consumption of large quantities of alcohol has a range of detrimental physical and emotional effects on your body.

Magnesium is a mineral with a profoundly calming effect on the nervous system and muscles of the body. Magnesium deficiency is extremely common and when you are stressed, your body uses up and excretes large quantities of magnesium. People who take magnesium regularly report feeling more relaxed, coping with stress better and having deeper, more restful sleep. Magnesium is available in powder or tablet form.

Improve your time management. Feeling like you don't have enough time to get things done is one of the most common sources of stress. It is important to learn how to prioritize urgent tasks and unpleasant tasks, so that you make the time to get them done first. This will give you peace of mind and help you to feel more relaxed. The website www.lifehack.org offers plenty of tips on how to be more productive and less stressed.

Make time for your favorite leisure activities. Many people have a fun deficiency in their lives. So much of our life is taken up by duties and responsibilities, that there is often little time left over for fun recreational activities. Don't neglect your hobbies or the important people in your life. Make time for those activities you are passionate about and make time for the people in your life who make you laugh.

Assess your communication skills. Relationship problems are a common source of stress, whether they are personal or work relationships. Often the problems stem from poor communication skills. Developing active listening skills and an assertive speaking manner can help to make your interactions with others more positive, and reduce the risk of misunderstandings. There are books and courses available to help you with this topic, or you can see a counsellor for personalized help. An excellent counsellor we recommend is Wendy Perkins. Her website is www.couragetochange.com.au Wendy does telephone counselling.

Foods to eliminate from your diet

Modern diets are typically high in sugar, starch and fat. This is a recipe for immune system dysfunction, chronic inflammation and generative disease; not to mention nutritional deficiencies. The foods listed below are capable of irritating the lining of your digestive tract, thus making it more permeable and creating what is known as leaky gut syndrome. This condition is thought to be the origin of all allergies and autoimmune disease.

Eliminating the following foods from your diet will greatly help your immune system and your digestive system. Approximately 70 to 80 percent of the immune cells in your body are in your digestive tract. Every time you consume a food that you are intolerant to or cannot digest adequately, it triggers an immune reaction inside your digestive tract. This produces inflammation and tissue destruction. When the digestive lining becomes too porous (leaky), undigested food molecules, bacteria, fungi, yeast and bacterial toxins can gain entry into your bloodstream. These toxins first flood your liver, and then travel throughout your body. This creates systemic toxicity.

The following foods need to be eliminated from your diet:

Gluten and dairy products

Everyone with an autoimmune disease, or allergies or food intolerance needs to avoid these foods all the time. They are difficult to digest, promote increased intestinal permeability and can trigger the production of auto-antibodies and subsequent development of autoimmune disease. Even if you do not have any known immune system problems, we recommend all women avoid gluten and dairy products for at least three months before conception, and right throughout pregnancy. These foods can promote excess mucus production in the fallopian tubes and they can make your cervical mucus less hospitable to sperm. They may also increase the risk of pre-eclampsia. We recommend all men with anti-sperm antibodies, or autoimmune disease or allergies avoid gluten and dairy products.

Gluten is found in the following grains: wheat, rye, oats, barley, spelt and kamut. Gluten is also hidden in many processed foods under another name, such as maltodextrin, starch or dextrose. Read food labels carefully and avoid everything that contains gluten. In susceptible people, consuming gluten triggers the production of inflammatory chemicals by immune cells called cytokines. You do not need to have celiac disease to experience health problems from eating gluten. If you want to follow a gluten free diet you must do it fully and consistently to experience the improvements. There's no going on and off the diet.

There are plenty of gluten free foods available such as gluten free bread, breakfast cereals, pasta, crackers, biscuits, etcetera. Many of these are gluten free junk food and are not suitable as part of a pre-conception diet. Grains are rapidly digested into glucose (sugar) once you ingest them and sugar promotes inflammation. Sugar also feeds pathogenic bacteria in the intestines, as well as Candida, yeast and fungi. Grains are acid forming, meaning their breakdown products increase the level of acidity in your body. Fruits and vegetables are alkaline. Small amounts of gluten free grains are acceptable occasionally, but it is best to base your diet on protein and vegetables.

Dairy products also need to be avoided and that means cow's milk and everything that contains cow's milk. It is the protein in milk that is harmful to the immune system; the protein is called casein. The lactose in milk is not a problem unless you are lactose intolerant. Therefore avoid all cow's milk, including lactose free milk. Some people can tolerate dairy products made from goat, sheep or water buffalo milk; this depends on the state of your immune system and digestive system. For now please avoid those dairy products too. There are plenty of excellent sources of calcium besides dairy products.

Foods high in calcium

- Bones in canned salmon and sardines
- Green leafy vegetables such as bok choy, kale and broccoli
- Tahini
- Nuts and seeds
- Figs
- Legumes

You can take a calcium supplement if you wish, but most cases of osteoporosis are not caused by inadequate calcium intake. They are caused by vitamin D deficiency, magnesium deficiency and conditions that cause excess calcium to be lost from the skeleton. You do not need to consume any dairy products to obtain sufficient calcium; dairy products cause far more harm to most people's health than benefits.

Avoid processed vegetable oil and margarine

The majority of vegetable oil sold in the supermarket is highly refined (meaning the antioxidants and vitamins are missing) and processed in a way that damages the delicate fatty acids that make up the oil. Vegetable oil is typically extracted from seeds or nuts under high heat and conditions which expose the oil to oxygen and light; all of which damage the oil and promote the production of harmful substances called products of lipid peroxidation. Vegetable oil is a very recent addition to the human diet; these oils only came into widespread industrial production in the 1920s.

Please avoid corn, soy, cottonseed, safflower, sunflower, canola, peanut and sesame oil, and all foods containing these oils. All of those oils are high in the omega 6 fatty acid linoleic acid. In your body linoleic acid is converted into arachidonic acid, which is a building block for highly inflammatory chemicals. These oils have no nutritional benefits to your body and in fact they are responsible for free radical damage inside your body when you consume them. Your body actually uses up its own antioxidant stores to metabolize these oils. The only beneficial vegetable oils are extra virgin, cold pressed olive oil and macadamia nut oil and organic coconut oil. Olive and macadamia nut oils are high in monounsaturated fats, which are far more heat stable and less prone to oxidation. Coconut oil is high in saturated fat, which is even more stable.

Deep fried takeaway food and fried snack foods usually contain trans fatty acids. These are abnormally shaped fats that your body doesn't really know how to use. These fats are inflammation promoters, plus they increase your risk of heart disease, strokes and cancer. Avoid food that has the words "vegetable oil" in the ingredient list, and particularly avoid "partially hydrogenated vegetable oil".

Avoid all margarine; even margarine free of trans fatty acids. It doesn't matter whether the margarine was made of nuts, seeds or olive oil; the creation of a spreadable texture damages the delicate fats and makes the product harmful. Margarine is high in omega 6 fats, which promote inflammation.

Avoid sugar

Sugar acts as a fertilizer for bad bacteria, yeast and fungi in your digestive tract. Sugar suppresses your immune system and leaves you less capable of fighting off infections. It also creates inflammation and free radical damage in your body. Foods with a high glycemic index (breakfast cereal, most bread, soft drinks, potatoes, rice) are rapidly digested into sugar. The rise in blood sugar promotes the release of insulin by your pancreas. High insulin levels raise inflammation. High sugar diets can inhibit ovulation because sugar promotes insulin secretion. Sugar is especially harmful to women with polycystic ovarian syndrome. Avoid adding sugar to tea or coffee; stevia and xylitol are both suitable natural sugar substitutes. Avoid fruit juice, as it is so concentrated that it has a similar effect in your body to soft drinks. Sugar is addictive and it promotes mood swings, therefore it isn't always easy to eliminate sugar from your diet. Taking a chromium and magnesium supplement will make you less likely to crave sugar.

Avoid processed red meat

Avoid deli meat such as ham, bacon, hotdogs, sausages (organic, preservative free are fine), smoked and corned meat. These foods promote inflammation and the preservative they contain (sodium nitrite) promotes stomach cancer. Also avoid charred meat. The healthiest cooking method is cooking in water; such as soup, stew, casseroles and steaming. Oven roasting is okay if there is some water present in the roasting tray. Frying, grilling and particularly char grilling promote the production of heterocyclic amines, which are carcinogenic.

Avoid alcohol

You need to avoid alcohol for several reasons. Alcohol promotes leaky gut syndrome, intestinal inflammation and it promotes the growth of yeast and fungi in the intestinal tract. Alcohol also depletes your body of several nutrients.

Avoid food additives

Avoid all artificial colors, flavours, preservatives and artificial sweeteners. Many are known to cause cancer and increase the risk of birth defects. Food additives are easy to avoid if you don't eat processed foods.

Avoid everything you are allergic or intolerant to

The foods most likely to cause allergic type reactions in the body are dairy products (particularly cow's milk), gluten, wheat, soy, yeast, oranges, nuts, eggs and shellfish. You may have other food sensitivities and these can be determined with the help of your naturopath or nutritionist. Even foods that are supposedly healthy will harm you if you are allergic or intolerant to them.

Other strategies for reducing inflammation

Be careful how you cook

Some cooking methods promote the formation of highly inflammatory chemicals called advanced glycation end products (AGEs). High heat and prolonged cooking time are the biggest culprits. Therefore fried food, grilled food, burnt food and deep fried food is high in these compounds. The foods highest in AGEs include bacon, pizza, fried chicken, fried eggs, hot chips, fried fish, char grilled meat, fried potatoes and burnt toast. AGEs increase the production of an inflammatory chemical called C-reactive protein in your body, as well as a host of other chemicals that over stimulate your immune system. AGEs can also form in your own body if you have high blood sugar, (such as diabetes or insulin resistance), or after you eat sugar. AGEs cause free radical damage to the proteins in your body and this will age you more quickly. The healthiest cooking methods use water, such as steaming, poaching and cooking soups, stews and casseroles.

Resolve chronic infections

Chronic infections greatly increase the level of inflammation in your body. Viral, bacterial or fungal infections are often hidden because they cause subtle symptoms that are not obviously related to an infection. Chronic infections can make you feel tired and run down and can make your energy levels fluctuate. You may have good days and good weeks, when your immune system is starting to get on top of the infection, but then your immune system is weakened and you feel tired and run down again.

Nutrient deficiencies, stress, poor quality or quantity sleep and a high sugar intake are the most common factors that weaken your immune system. If you become infected with a microbe, your immune system may not have the resources to overcome the infection. The inflammatory chemicals your immune cells make in order to try and overcome the infection increase inflammation, free radical damage and wear and tear on your body. Resolving the infection is vital for reducing inflammation. See chapter 6 for strategies for overcoming infections.

9. Environmental Chemicals and Infertility

Environmental chemicals are thought to play a major role in the escalating rates of infertility seen in the last 50 years. We believe environmental chemicals are a leading cause of menstrual cycle abnormalities, hormone disorders, sperm abnormalities and miscarriage. We believe they are a major contributor to what is commonly referred to as unexplained infertility, and problems that many doctors refer to as genetic. Environmental chemicals are capable of causing genetic problems, and they are particularly harmful if you are deficient in certain key nutrients; particularly vitamin D, selenium and B vitamins.

In this chapter we will outline which particular chemicals are strongly linked to infertility and give you suggestions on how to reduce your exposure to them. It is impossible to avoid these chemicals entirely, and it is not necessary. This chapter of the book can seem quite depressing because nearly every substance we come into contact with in modern life contains a chemical that can harm us in some way. However, there are many easy ways you can reduce your exposure to these chemicals, while maintaining your current lifestyle. Also it is important to remember that the healthier you are, the better your diet, and the better your organs of elimination (particularly your liver), the less likely you are to be harmed by environmental chemicals.

Since the second half of the 20th century, more than 80 thousand man made synthetic chemicals have been released into the environment. They range from plastics and pesticides to detergents and cosmetics. These new chemicals were never a part of the environment our great grandparents lived in, but now we can detect measurable quantities in our water, air, soil, food, and even our own bodies. All new pharmaceutical drugs that are released into the market must go through fairly rigorous testing; however in the majority of cases, when it comes to the chemical industry, there are no such requirements. New chemicals are simply not evaluated adequately for their potential risks to human health. Only if a product has been on the market for some time and there are concerns about its impact on health, will it undergo testing.

Unfortunately it is a fact that our economy relies very heavily on many of these chemicals, therefore governments are reluctant to dig deep and truly evaluate the harmful effects these chemicals are having on our lives. It is a sad fact that more than 85 percent of the more than 80 thousand registered synthetic chemicals have never been evaluated for their effects on human health. Even when chemicals are tested for safety; they are tested in isolation. The reality is we are all exposed to a plethora of chemicals at the same time, which have an additive effect.

Which chemicals have harmful effects on fertility?

Many of the chemicals that adversely affect fertility do so because they disrupt the body's hormone balance. Chemicals of this nature are referred to as endocrine disruptors. Endocrine glands are hormone producing glands; such as the ovaries, testes, thyroid gland and others. The official definition of an endocrine disruptor is:

"An endogenous agent that interferes with the synthesis, secretion, transport, binding, action or elimination of natural hormones in the body that are responsible for the maintenance of homeostasis, reproduction, development and/or behaviour".[99]

A wide range of chemicals fit the definition of endocrine disruptor, including heavy metals, pesticides, plasticizers, prescription medication, radiation and organic solvents.

Who is most at risk of chemical exposure?

Some people are far more likely to accumulate harmful levels of chemicals in their bodies than others. Your occupation is one major determining factor. People in the following occupations are most susceptible:

- Dentists and dental assistants
- Veterinarians
- People who work in the dry cleaning industry
- Non-organic farmers
- Clothing industry
- Cleaners
- Cosmetics industry
- Laboratory workers
- Plastics industry
- Factory workers
- Mechanics
- Painters
- Welders
- Metal workers

As a generalization, men are more likely to be exposed to harmful chemicals through their occupation than women. Most women use a far greater amount of personal care products, toiletries and cleaning products than men. These, combined with cosmetics expose some women to very high levels of harmful chemicals. We will now go through the environmental chemicals that are most strongly implicated in infertility, and give you suggestions on how to minimize your exposure.

Phthalates

Phthalates are chemicals used as lubricants, solvents, plasticizers and stabilizers. They are added to plastic to make it softer and more flexible. They have been around since the 1930s and are now widely distributed throughout the environment.

Where are they found?

- Children's toys, particularly soft plastic chew toys for infants
- Some sex toys
- Nail polish
- Hair spray
- Most paint (in the solvent)
- Most lipstick, where they are used to make it glossy
- Most perfume

- Many skin moisturizers, cleansers, shampoo and other personal care products
- Air fresheners
- Vinyl shower curtains
- Rubber thongs
- Soft PET plastic water bottles
- Medical tubing and medical plastic bags

Phthalates can be absorbed through your skin, ingested, or inhaled in polluted air.

Adverse health effects of phthalates

Phthalates have the ability to reduce luteinizing hormone production, increase follicle stimulating hormone production and delay ovulation. They can also impair your body's ability to manufacture sex hormones.[100] Phthalates interfere with the action of insulin in your body, therefore make weight loss much more difficult. Phthalates are implicated as one cause of worldwide declining sperm counts.

Phthalates mimic the actions of estrogen in your body, therefore pregnant women exposed to high levels of phthalates are more likely to give birth to sons with genital abnormalities. These include undescended testes (cryptorchidism) and hypospadias (where the opening of the penis is on the shaft, rather than on the tip). Boys with those conditions are at higher risk of testicular cancer in adulthood. Phthalates are also thought to contribute to early puberty in children.

Recommendations for minimizing exposure to phthalates

- Minimize the use of plastic water bottles and food storage containers. Particularly avoid keeping oily foods in any plastic containers, as fat is able to draw plastic molecules from the container and into your food. Use glass, ceramic and stainless steel containers instead.
- Never eat hot food or drink hot liquids out of plastic containers. Heat promotes the migration of plastic into food.
- Avoid using cling wrap, particularly if it comes into contact with food.
- Don't give plastic teething rings or chew toys to infants. Use wooden toys or rusks instead.

- Many cosmetics and personal care products contain phthalates, as a component of the fragrance. Therefore it is best to purchase fragrance free products. Fortunately there are now several brands of entirely natural cosmetics and personal care products that are free of phthalates and other undesirables.
- Avoid using air freshener in your home. Get rid of the source of odor instead and use pure essential oils to fragrance your home.

In 1999 the European Union banned the use of phthalates in some products, including baby toys. In Canada and the USA the chemicals have been removed from infant bottle nipples and other products designed to go in a baby's mouth. At this stage phthalates have not been banned in Australia.

Bisphenol A (BPA)

Bisphenol A is the building block of polycarbonate plastic. It makes plastic hard, translucent and shatter resistant. It is also used in the manufacture of epoxy resins. Globally approximately six billion pounds of bisphenol A are used by industry each year.

Where is it found?

Polycarbonate plastic is usually hard, translucent plastic that has the recycling number 7 on it. Large plastic water bottles that sit on top of cooling dispensers usually contain bisphenol A. Small, hard sports and camping water bottles also usually contain this compound. Many types of plastic baby bottles contain bisphenol A, as do many plastic storage containers. Bisphenol A is found in the white resin lining of some canned foods such as tinned tomatoes, beetroot and baked beans. Increased temperatures (cooking and sterilization) and storage cause increased leaching of bisphenol A into food. Bisphenol A is also found in dental sealants and the lining of some milk containers.

Adverse health effects of bisphenol A

Bisphenol A binds to the estrogen receptors in your body and has a strong estrogenic effect. The Centers for Disease Control in the USA have detected bisphenol A in the urine of close to

93 percent of 2,517 people aged six years and older. Females had much higher levels than males.[101] Research has shown that bisphenol A interferes with sex hormone production. Women with polycystic ovarian syndrome appear to be more sensitive to the effects of this chemical than healthy women.

BPA makes it harder to lose weight because it interferes with the release of a hormone that regulates body weight called adiponectin.[102] A study measured bisphenol A levels in women undergoing IVF. There was a trend towards higher levels in women who did not become pregnant. Unfortunately, exposure to BPA is associated with miscarriage and the presence of antinuclear antibodies.[103] These antibodies are a feature of several autoimmune diseases; therefore BPA seems to increase the risk of developing autoimmune disease. In males BPA can increase the size of the prostate gland and impair sperm production.

In 2003 scientists at the Case Western Reserve University in the USA made a startling discovery. They were studying eggs (oocytes) in mice when they noticed high rates of chromosome abnormalities inside the eggs. The chromosome abnormalities are called aneuploidy, which means either a loss or gain of chromosomes inside a cell as a result of an error in cell division. In humans aneuploidy can cause miscarriage or birth defects, including Down syndrome. Eventually the scientists made the discovery. They had been using harsh detergents to wash the animals' polycarbonate plastic cages and water bottles. The harsh detergents had damaged the plastic and caused bisphenol A to leach out of the plastic cages and water bottles. Exposure to this chemical was what caused the mouse eggs to contain a dramatically high number of chromosome abnormalities.[104]

Recommendations for minimizing exposure to bisphenol A

- Minimize your intake of canned foods. Most canned soup, stew, fruit and vegetables contain large quantities of bisphenol A if the can they are in has a white resin lining. Buy fresh or frozen vegetables instead.
- Minimize drinking out of plastic water bottles. Install a water filer on your tap and store water in glass bottles.

- Avoid plastic baby bottles; use glass instead. Some plastic is free of BPA, which is better, but glass is still preferable.
- Don't eat hot food or drink hot liquids out of plastic containers.
- Avoid using cling wrap and never microwave food that has been covered in it.
- Avoid plastic cutlery
- If you use a plastic lunch box, do not place it in a dishwasher. The high temperature and harsh chemicals cause the plastic to break down and leach more bisphenol A into your food. Throw away plastic containers that start to look worn.
- Avoid using plastic containers with the recycling number 7 on them, as in most cases they contain bisphenol A.
- Avoid drinking hot liquids out of Styrofoam cups, or cardboard cups that have a plastic lining. Drink coffee and tea out of ceramic mugs or glass instead.
- When you are pregnant, make sure you take a folic acid supplement, and eat plenty of green leafy vegetables, which are rich in folic acid. A study conducted at Duke University in the USA found that folic acid helps to protect fetuses from some of the harmful effects of bisphenol A.[105]

Parabens

Parabens are antimicrobial preservatives used in food, medicines, cosmetics and personal care products. Parabens applied to your skin are absorbed into your bloodstream. Parabens accumulate in your body and are stored in body fat and breasts (which are mostly fat). Therefore, the longer you have been alive and using parabens, the more you will have in your body.

Where are they found?

There are several types of parabens: methylparaben, ethylparaben, propylparaben and butylparaben. Have a look at your toiletries and you'll be surprised how often these terms are mentioned on the label. Parabens are found widely in shampoo and conditioner, deodorant, moisturizer, toothpaste, shaving lotions, personal lubricants, sunscreen, foundation, fake tan, liquid medication and many other places.

Adverse health effects of parabens

Parabens are estrogen mimics and have the ability to bind to estrogen receptors in your body. In this way, they worsen all hormonal conditions caused by estrogen dominance, such as endometriosis and uterine fibroids. Parabens aggravate the symptoms of progesterone deficiency. They have been linked to breast cancer, infertility, abnormal fetal development and sperm abnormalities. Luckily many personal care products are available that are entirely free of parabens. Read labels carefully.

Organochlorine compounds

Organochlorine compounds include DDT and related compounds that were widely used as pesticides in Australia. The majority of these pesticides have been banned in recent years. Examples of organochlorine pesticides include aldrin, chlordane, dieldrin, endrin, heptachlor and lindane. They were widely used to control termites and protect wood from other pests, and also used as fungicides and herbicides. Unfortunately, most of these compounds are extremely persistent in the environment. They take a long time to break down and they accumulate in body fat. Therefore we are all still exposed to these compounds, predominantly through the consumption of animal products, water, airborne exposure and breast milk.

Adverse health effects of organochlorine compounds

The following adverse health outcomes have been linked to organochlorine exposure in women and men:

Females

- Infertility
- Impaired ovulation
- Impaired sex hormone production
- Altered function of the endometrium (lining of the uterus)
- Miscarriage
- Impaired fetal development

Males

- Infertility
- Poor semen quality
- Increased risk of birth defects
- Miscarriage[106, 107]

Recommendations for minimizing exposure to organochlorine compounds

Organic foods are lower in these compounds than conventional produce, particularly animal foods. Therefore, if available and affordable, try to purchase organic meat, poultry and eggs. Avoid farmed fish. Avoid eating the skin of poultry and fatty cuts of meat because these compounds are fat soluble, therefore highest levels are found in the fat of animals. Avoid offal.

Dioxins

Dioxins are some of the most widespread chemicals in the world today. Every human body, including every newborn contains measurable levels of dioxins. Dioxin is a general term that describes a range of chemicals that are formed during the incineration of plastic and industrial compounds; from industrial processes that use chlorine (such as bleaching), and during the combustion of diesel and gasoline. According to the US Environmental Protection Agency, there is no safe level of dioxin exposure and they are a known human carcinogen (cancer causing agent). The problem with dioxins is they break down extremely slowly; therefore they accumulate in soil, in fish, poultry and meat, and us.

Dioxins are endocrine disruptors, capable of causing hormonal disorders and increasing the risk of endometriosis, uterine fibroids and breast cancer. Studies done on monkeys have shown that adult monkeys exposed to dioxins develop endometriosis, and when endometrial cells are implanted into monkeys, dioxins stimulate their growth. It is difficult to avoid dioxins because they are so widespread in our environment, however by choosing organic animal foods such as meat, poultry and eggs, you will reduce your exposure. Dioxins are formed during chlorine bleaching, therefore do not use chlorine bleached tissues, toilet paper, tampons, paper cups, or any other products that come in contact with your body. Buy non-chlorine bleached paper for printing and photo-copying.

Organic solvents

People who work in the clothing, paint and plastic industries are most likely to be exposed to organic solvents. Some health care professionals and laboratory workers are also exposed. Organic solvents can impair both female and male fertility, but they seem to have more effects in women. Research has shown that exposure to organic solvents increases the length of time it takes a woman to fall pregnant;[108] increases the risk of miscarriage and increases the risk of major malformations in the fetus 13 fold.[109]

Flame retardants

Brominated flame retardants are a group of chemicals used on a wide range of household items to reduce their tendency to catch fire. Flame retardants are used on carpets, mattresses, furniture, clothing, computers, televisions, cables, CD players, mobile phones, the interior of cars and many other items. The problem is the flame retardants out-gas from these items and are then inhaled or ingested by you.

Flame retardants have also been found in animal foods; therefore you will ingest them through your diet. Flame retardants are very slow to break down, and they accumulate in body fat. In 2004 the Australian Department of Environment and Heritage conducted studies on the levels of flame retardants in blood samples taken from Australians. Levels were found to be not as high as in North Americans, but higher than in Europeans and Asians.

Flame retardants are endocrine disruptors. Some act as estrogen mimics and some mimic T4 thyroid hormone; having the ability to bind to T4 receptor sites. Animal studies have found flame retardants to cause structural changes in ovaries and impair sperm function. A Swedish study conducted on humans found an increased risk of testicular cancer in sons of women with high blood levels of flame retardants. A Danish-Finish study found concentrations of flame retardants to be higher in the breast milk of women who had sons with cryptorchidism (un-descended testes).[110]

Recommendations for reducing exposure to flame retardants

It is not possible to avoid exposure to flame retardants because they are present in so many items we come in contact with each day. However, research has shown that the main form of exposure to these compounds is through inhalation and ingestion of house dust. Therefore, you can reduce exposure by keeping dust levels in your home to a minimum. It is also important to open the windows in your house and ensure good ventilation. The levels of indoor air pollution in most homes are far higher than outdoor air pollution.

Glycol ether

Glycol ether is used in printing inks, surface coatings, some cosmetics, cleaning products, some pesticides and as flow improvers in water-based paint. Research carried out in the UK found that exposure to glycol ether reduced sperm motility in men attending infertility clinics.[111]

Perfluorochemicals

These are a group of chemicals used to make Teflon and other non-stick cooking pans, as well as Scotchguard and stain and water repellent products. They are used on carpets, curtains and some clothing. They are used in the inner lining of microwave popcorn bags, and some takeaway food containers and packaging that might come in contact with grease. Research has linked these chemicals to immune disorders, cancer and infertility. Research conducted at the University of California, Los Angeles found that women with higher levels of perfluorochemicals in their bodies are more likely to have menstrual problems and take longer to conceive. It is safest to use stainless steel or cast iron cookware. If you do use non-stick cookware, you must cook at low temperatures only, as high heat will release more of these chemicals from the pans.

Heavy metals and infertility

Several heavy metals can impair your fertility if you have abnormally high levels in your body. In men, lead, mercury, cobalt and cadmium can impair sperm production and cause testicular damage. Men most at risk are those who do metal work, welding, or work in ammunitions manufacture. Exposure to lead can occur in the paint industry. In general, men are more at risk of heavy metal toxicity affecting their fertility than women.

Lead

In women, even low levels of lead increase the risk of miscarriage and stillbirth. During pregnancy lead can leach from your bones and cross the placenta to adversely affect the development of your fetus. Most of the time people develop lead toxicity because they live in a mining or industrial town. Lead may also be present in electrical wiring, contaminated soil, old roofing and plumbing. Lead is present in old paint, which you can become exposed to during renovations.

Symptoms of lead toxicity include fatigue, microcytic anemia (small red blood cells), high blood pressure, cognitive impairment, loss of appetite and muscle pain. If you are concerned about heavy metal toxicity, see page 194 for information on hair mineral analysis.

The following nutrients will help to detoxify your body from lead:

Zinc and calcium are antagonistic to lead; therefore increasing your intake of these minerals will reduce the amount of lead you absorb from your environment.

Selenium binds to lead directly and can help to remove it from your body.

Magnesium, iron, vitamin C and vitamin D. Deficiency of any of these nutrients increases the amount of lead you absorb through your gastrointestinal tract.

Mercury

Mercury toxicity is linked to infertility and miscarriage. In men, excess mercury affects sperm quality and quantity. It is vitally important not to have high levels of mercury in your body when you fall pregnant, because it would enter your baby's circulation and impair the development of its nervous system. Mercury is released into the air through industrial pollution. Mercury then enters oceans and rivers, where it is converted to methylmercury. Fish ingest methylmercury and it builds up in their bodies. As a general rule, the bigger and older the fish is, the more mercury is inside its body. If you regularly eat this kind of fish, mercury will accumulate in your body over time. Dental amalgams are the other most common source of mercury ingestion. Women with high body levels of mercury are at risk of giving birth to infants with birth defects and neurological impairments, and autistic children.

Fish to avoid

The following fish are highest in mercury and should be avoided entirely by women and men prior to conception and during pregnancy:

- billfish (swordfish / broadbill and marlin)
- shark/flake
- orange roughy (sea perch)
- catfish

Canned tuna is not particularly high in mercury, but most of it is caught from highly polluted waters. We recommend a brand of canned fish called Fish 4 Ever which you can purchase from health food stores, or see their website at www.fish-4-ever.com

The following nutrients will help to detoxify your body from mercury:

Selenium is an antagonist to mercury. In most instances people with high levels of mercury in their body are selenium deficient. We recommend a supplement of 200 micrograms of selenomethionine per day.

Zinc is also an antagonist to mercury. The recommended dose is 20 to 40 milligrams daily.

Coriander, chlorella and alpha lipoic acid are chelating agents that help to remove mercury from your body.

Cadmium

Cadmium is a by-product of the mining and smelting of zinc and lead. It is used in nickel-cadmium batteries, paint pigments and PVC plastic. Cadmium is found in many insecticides, fungicides and fertilizers; in fact the most widely used fertilizer in many parts of the world, Superphosphate is high in cadmium. Cadmium is also present in cigarettes, motor oil and exhaust. You inhale much of the cadmium that gets inside your body. Alcohol consumption increases the gastrointestinal absorption of cadmium into your body.

Cadmium has a particularly destructive effect on sperm production. Cadmium toxicity has been strongly linked with male infertility; it impairs sperm production and increases sperm abnormalities.

Environmental chemicals and infertility: not limited to humans

A relationship between environmental contaminants and reproductive disorders has been observed in nearly every species of animal on the planet; from fish and seagulls, to polar bears, alligators, seals and frogs. The brilliant book *Our Stolen Future* describes the known effects of environmental pollutants on birth defects, sexual abnormalities and reproductive failure in wildlife and humans. Scientists have known about the devastating effects of environmental chemicals on the ability of wildlife to reproduce for many decades. Humans are really just another animal on this planet, therefore it would be naive to think the same won't happen to us. If you are interested in reading more about the harmful effects of environmental chemicals on fertility, see the website www.ourstolenfuture.com

10. Essential tests for the investigation of female infertility

This chapter will outline the medical tests you may need to have in order to determine the cause of your infertility. Many of the tests are standard and your doctor may have already performed them. Some of the tests may not be applicable to you, while other tests are vitally important, but your doctor may have overlooked them. We will describe blood tests first, and then other investigations.

Blood tests

Hormone tests

The following sex hormones should be tested. This is particularly relevant for women with very short menstrual cycles (21 to 25 days) or very long menstrual cycles (32 to 42 days). In general, having a short menstrual cycle may be an indicator of declining ovarian reserve (diminishing number of eggs in the ovaries). Women with longer cycles often have good ovarian reserve and they usually have more fertile years left.

FSH (follicle stimulating hormone)

Should be tested on day 2 or 3 of your menstrual cycle (day 1 is the first day of bleeding)

Normal range: 2 - 20 U/L

FSH is made in the pituitary gland of your brain and it stimulates the ovaries to manufacture estrogen. As a woman gets closer to menopause, FSH levels rise. An FSH test is one indicator of ovarian reserve; basically telling you how many good eggs you have left and how many more fertile years you have before you reach menopause. An FSH level under 6 is considered excellent, while a level greater than 13 often indicates diminishing ovarian reserve. The ratio of FSH to LH (luteinizing hormone) should be close to 1:1. If the level of LH is significantly higher, this may indicate polycystic ovarian syndrome. Recently it has been discovered that a test for anti-mullerian hormone is a more precise indicator of ovarian reserve than FSH. This test will be explained later in this chapter.

LH (Luteinizing hormone)

Should be tested on day 2 or 3.

Normal range: Less than 7 U/L

Luteinizing hormone should be low at this phase of your menstrual cycle. A high level may indicate polycystic ovarian syndrome.

Oestradiol (E2)

This is the main form of estrogen in your body and the strongest form of estrogen. Your ovaries manufacture oestradiol in response to stimulation from FSH. This test should be performed on day 2 or 3 of your cycle and the normal range at this stage is 100 – 200 pmol/L (27 - 54 pg/mL).

Progesterone

Progesterone should be tested on day 21 of a 28 day menstrual cycle. Women with a regular cycle that is 28 days or close to it are generally assumed to be ovulating. Not every woman has a 28 day cycle of course; therefore you need to have the progesterone blood test 7 days before your next menstrual period begins. This is because the follicular phase (first half) of the menstrual cycle can vary in length quite a bit, but the luteal phase (second half) tends to be a fixed length. If you have been charting your menstrual cycle on a calendar, you should know when seven days before your next period should be. Progesterone needs to be tested in the mid-luteal phase. In women with irregular menstrual cycles or long cycles, it may be necessary to have a progesterone blood test each week in order to establish if ovulation has occurred. Women with cycles more than 42 days apart are unlikely to be ovulating regularly.

A mid-luteal progesterone level greater than 25 nmol/L (7.8 ng/mL) indicates the formation of a corpus luteum after ovulation. Therefore you have ovulated, but sometimes the corpus luteum cannot sustain progesterone production or levels do not rise high enough to maintain a pregnancy. Progesterone supplementation is vital for women who fall into that category. Have your progesterone blood test done in the morning. Progesterone levels may drop up to fifty percent by the afternoon, and after a meal.

Progesterone levels during pregnancy

While you are pregnant, your progesterone level needs to steadily climb. The following ranges indicate the normal progesterone levels during the three trimesters of pregnancy:

1st trimester.. 30 - 100 nmol/L (9 - 31 ng/mL)

2nd trimester.. 110 - 340 nmol/L (35 - 107 ng/mL)

3rd trimester .... 210 - 600 nmol/L (66 - 189 ng/mL)

Prolactin

Prolactin is made by the pituitary gland in the brain. It stimulates the breasts to produce milk, therefore prolactin levels become very high after childbirth. However, it is normal to have some prolactin in your bloodstream all the time. This test should be performed on day 2 or 3 of your cycle and your prolactin should be less than 500 mIU/L.

Elevated prolactin can suppress ovulation. Women with high prolactin often get breast pain before their period and experience PMS. Sometimes prolactin levels fluctuate, and only become elevated at night. This can make the blood test not a reliable indicator. Some women with polycystic ovarian syndrome have elevated prolactin. If your level is significantly elevated, you may need to have an MRI scan of your brain to check for a pituitary tumor. These tumors are tiny, they do not spread throughout the body and they are easily managed.

Cortisol

Cortisol is made by your adrenal glands and is produced in response to stress. High levels of cortisol can indicate extreme or long term stress and excess cortisol has a negative effect on fertility. High cortisol is often seen in those with insulin resistance (syndrome X), polycystic ovarian syndrome and women who carry excess weight in their abdominal area.

Cortisol should be tested in the morning; approximately 7:30 am to 8:30 am at any phase of your menstrual cycle.

Morning cortisol should be between 200 and 650 nmol/L (7.25 and 23.56 ug/dL). Afternoon cortisol should be between 100 and 400 nmol/L (3.62 and 14.50 ug/dL).

DHEA-S

Dehydroepiandrosterone sulphate is made in your adrenal glands. The hormone has immune system benefits and improves energy levels and stamina. However it is a male hormone and high levels are often seen in women with polycystic ovarian syndrome.

The normal range for women is 1-11 μmol/L

Free testosterone

Your ovaries and adrenal glands manufacture testosterone. Free testosterone refers to the active testosterone in your bloodstream that is not bound to a carrier protein.

Your free testosterone level should be less than 4 pmol/L. Women with polycystic ovarian syndrome typically have raised levels.

Free Androgen Index (FAI)

Androgens are all the male hormones in your body; testosterone and others. In women the free androgen index should be between 1 and 8 percent. Women with polycystic ovarian syndrome typically have raised levels, and this test is very helpful in the diagnosis of PCOS.

Anti-mullerian hormone (AMH)

Your level of anti-mullerian hormone is a good indicator of your ovarian reserve. Ovarian reserve is a term used to describe the number of good quality eggs left within your ovaries. You are born with approximately two million eggs, and during your lifetime your eggs decline as they are lost through ovulation and natural cell death. You only lose approximately 400 eggs through ovulation; the rest are lost through cell death. The rate at which women lose eggs varies enormously, and that accounts for the variation in age that women experience menopause. Cigarette smoking, poor diet and stress are known to speed up the rate of egg loss, while having a nutrient rich diet and taking good care of your health can prolong the life of your eggs.

Anti-mullerian hormone is produced by immature eggs in your ovaries that wake up from their dormant state and develop into mature eggs. Specifically it is the granulosa cells of early developing follicles that produce this hormone. As time goes by and you start to run out of follicles, your blood level of anti-mullerian hormone will also decline. Women with a family history of early menopause, severe endometriosis, autoimmune disease or a history of surgery to the ovaries are all at risk of early menopause and should have an AMH blood test. Women with diminished ovarian reserve find it harder to fall pregnant and they are at higher risk of miscarriage. This is probably because older eggs are more likely to contain chromosome abnormalities. Your level of anti-mullerian hormone does not fluctuate a great deal during your menstrual cycle; therefore you can have this blood test at any time.

Women with an AMH level greater than 14 pmol/L have a higher ovarian reserve and better chance of conception. A very high reading may indicate polycystic ovarian syndrome. Even if you have healthy, young eggs in your ovaries, several other factors can stand in the way of conception (such as blocked tubes); therefore this blood test should not be relied upon too heavily. This test is not covered by Medicare; it costs approximately $60.

Thyroid blood tests

Even a subtle thyroid disorder can drastically reduce your chance of conception; therefore all women should have a thorough thyroid blood test.

TSH (Thyroid Stimulating Hormone)

TSH is made by the pituitary gland in your brain and it stimulates your thyroid gland to manufacture hormones. A high TSH level can indicate an under active thyroid gland and a low TSH level can indicate an over active thyroid gland. Either scenario can impair your fertility.

Ideally your TSH level should be between 0.3 and 2 mIU/L. Women are less likely to conceive and more likely to have a miscarriage if their TSH is above 2.5 mIU/L. If you have a diagnosed thyroid condition and are taking thyroid medication, you need your TSH level to be between 0.3 and 2 mIU/L. If it is not, you should speak to your doctor about adjusting your dose.

Free T4

T4 (thyroxine) is the main hormone produced by your thyroid gland. The normal range is 8 - 22 pmol/L (0.62 - 1.71 ng/dL).

Free T3

T3 (triiodothyronine) is the active thyroid hormone. Your body converts T4 into T3. Much of this conversion occurs in your liver.

The normal range is 2.5 - 6.0 pmol/L (162 - 390 pg/dL).

TSH during pregnancy

Your thyroid gland needs to pump out more hormones when you become pregnant. The following TSH levels are considered ideal during the three trimesters of pregnancy:

First trimester ....0.24 - 2.99 mIU/L

Second trimester ....0.46 - 2.95 mIU/L

Third trimester ....0.43 - 2.78 mIU/L[112]

Thyroid antibodies

It is very important to have a blood test to check for the presence of thyroid antibodies. This is especially important for women with immune system disorders such as autoimmune disease and allergies. Having thyroid antibodies in your bloodstream means your immune system is attacking your thyroid gland. The presence of thyroid antibodies indicates autoimmune thyroid disease: Hashimoto's thyroiditis, Graves' disease or autoimmune thyroiditis.

The normal ranges are as follows:

Anti-thyroglobulin abs ....less than 60 U/mL

Anti-thyroidal peroxidase abs ....less than 60 U/mL

TSH receptor antibodies

The presence of these antibodies is associated with Graves'

disease and Graves' eye disease. The normal range should be less than 1 IU/L.

Research has shown that women who test positive for thyroid antibodies are at increased risk of infertility, miscarriage, IVF failure, fetal death, pre-eclampsia, premature delivery, postpartum thyroiditis and postnatal depression.[113] If you test positive for thyroid antibodies it is vitally important that you follow our immune system guidelines in chapter 5.

Diabetes and metabolic blood tests

Having diabetes while pregnant raises the risk of giving birth to an excessively large baby, and thus increases the risk of delivery complications and the need for caesarean section. Diabetes also increases the risk of your baby being born with abnormally high body fat levels, and this increases the risk of obesity and cardiovascular disease in adulthood. High blood sugar while pregnant increases the risk of birth defects in your baby. Some women only develop diabetes while they are pregnant. This is called gestational diabetes.

Fasting blood glucose

A fasting blood glucose test is one way to detect the presence of diabetes. A normal fasting blood glucose level is 3.6 - 5.4 mmol/L (64 - 97 mg/dL).

Impaired glucose tolerance (or insulin resistance) is defined as a blood sugar of 5.5 - 6.9 mmol/L (99 - 124 mg/dL).

Diabetes is diagnosed if your blood sugar is above 6.9 mmol/L (124 mg/dL).

HbA1c test

This is also known as a glycated, or glycosylated haemoglobin test. It measures your average blood sugar for the previous three months. Specifically it measures how much glucose has been bound to your red blood cells for the previous three months. You do not have to fast before having this test.

A result of 6.5 percent or greater is considered to diagnose diabetes.

Glucose tolerance test

If your fasting blood sugar level is higher than ideal, but not high enough to be considered diabetic, you will usually be asked to have a glucose tolerance test. This measures your blood sugar level after you ingest a test dose of glucose (75 grams). Your blood sugar is tested over a period of two hours. It is best if your insulin levels are a lso tested along with glucose, therefore making this a glucose insulin tolerance test.

The normal values for a glucose tolerance test are below:

Time	Normal	Impaired glucose tolerance	Diabetes
Fasting	glucose 3.6 - 5.4 mmol/L (64 - 97 mg/dL) insulin below 10 mU/L	glucose 5.5 - 6.9 mmol/L (99 - 124 mg/dL) insulin above 10 mU/L	glucose >6.9 mmol/L (>124 mg/dL)
2 hours	glucose < 7.1 mmol/L (< 127 mg/dL) insulin 5 - 50 mU/L	glucose 7.2 - 11.0 mmol/L (129 - 198 mg/dL) insulin > 50 mU/L	glucose > 11mmol/L (> 198 mg/dL)

Serum insulin test

A high blood insulin level indicates insulin resistance or syndrome X. Women with insulin resistance are more likely to have ovulation problems, polycystic ovarian syndrome and be overweight. This is a fasting test. Your fasting level of insulin should be less than 10 mU/L.

Diagnosis of gestational diabetes

Gestational diabetes means diabetes during pregnancy. Elevated blood sugar while pregnant is dangerous for the health of your baby. Gestational diabetes typically starts in the 24th to 28th week of pregnancy. The test traditionally used to diagnose gestational diabetes is called a glucose challenge test. It involves drinking a 50 gram glucose solution and having a blood test one hour later. This is not a fasting test. A blood sugar level above 7.8 mmol/L (140 mg/dL) may indicate gestational diabetes.

A pregnant woman is considered to have gestational diabetes if her fasting blood glucose level is greater than 5.5 mmol/L (99mg/dL), or her two hour glucose tolerance test reveals a blood sugar level greater than 8 mmol/L (144mg/dL).

New recommendation for the diagnosis of gestational diabetes

As a result of recent research, a group of 50 international experts has determined that maternal blood glucose levels previously considered safe now pose a risk to mothers and their babies. As a result of five years of research conducted on more than 23 thousand pregnant women, plus the results of two other large trials, experts concluded that a fasting blood sugar level of 5.1 mmol/L (92mg/dL) or higher in a pregnant woman poses serious threats to mother and child. The current cut-off is 5.5 mmol/L (99mg/dL). According to Professor Jeremy Oats, of Melbourne's Royal Women's Hospital, under the new threshold, approximately 12 percent of pregnant Australian women have gestational diabetes.[114] This is worrying; you can read about the dangers of gestational diabetes on page 132. This is why it is so important to try and achieve a healthy weight and blood sugar level before you get pregnant, especially for women with polycystic ovarian syndrome. Trying to attain this while already pregnant is far more difficult.

Blood tests for nutrients

Vitamin D

All women must have a vitamin D blood test before attempting conception, as deficiency is so common. Vitamin D deficiency can inhibit ovulation, lead to hormone disorders and impair the health of your fetus if you do become pregnant.

The optimum blood level of 25 OH vitamin D is between 100 and 150 nmol/L (40 and 60 ng/mL).

Iron

A blood test called iron studies is the most thorough test of your body's iron status. Your blood iron level should be between 9 and 27 umol/L (50 and 150 ug/dL).

Your ferritin level is the amount of iron stored in your body, particularly your liver. It is a better indicator of your long term iron status. Your ferritin level should be between 20 and 160 ug/L.

Iodine

The iodine test is a urine test. Your doctor can arrange you to have this test performed at a local pathology company.

Your urinary iodine level must be between 100 and 300 micrograms per liter.

Red cell folate

This measures the amount of folate (folic acid) in your red blood cells. The normal level is greater than 630 nmol/L (278 ng/mL).

Serum vitamin B12

The normal amount of vitamin B12 to have in your bloodstream is 180 - 740 pmol/L (244 - 1003 pg/mL). Folate and vitamin B12 are vitally important for the development of your baby's nervous system and they help to protect the DNA inside your eggs and your partner's sperm from free radical damage.

Homocysteine blood test

This test is a useful indicator of how well you utilize folate and vitamin B12 in your body. If you are deficient in these B vitamins, or not utilizing them correctly, your blood homocysteine level will rise. Elevated homocysteine is related to an increased risk of heart attacks and strokes, female and male infertility, depression and an increased risk of having a child with autism.

Approximately 25 percent of the population have a mutation of the gene that is required for the conversion of homocysteine into the amino acid methionine. This leads to elevated homocysteine levels. The name of the enzyme that is required for the conversion is 5, 10-methylenetetrahydrofolate reductase. A test is available to check if you have this gene mutation; either a blood test or buccal swab (scraping the inner lining of your cheek). Women and men with this gene mutation have a higher risk of infertility. You may want to get this test performed if you have abnormally low blood folate or high blood homocysteine levels.

The normal level of homocysteine is 5 - 15 umol/L (0.67 - 2.02 mg/L).

Full blood count

This is a basic test that checks the health and quantity of your red and white blood cells. Too high or too low white blood cells indicate an immune system problem.

Blood tests for autoimmune disease

ANA (Anti-Nuclear Antibodies)

This is a non-specific test to check for the presence of autoimmune disease. More than 95 percent of patients with lupus test positive for anti-nuclear antibodies, but they are found in nearly all autoimmune disease. A positive anti-nuclear antibody test warrants further blood tests to check for the presence of other auto-antibodies.

DNA antibodies

This is a more specific blood test for systemic lupus erythematosus. In normal healthy people the level should be less than 5 IU/mL

Anti-DNA/Histone antibody.

If a woman reacts to the broken down DNA (histones) and it is a speckled pattern, then she is likely to mount an immune reaction to her own embryos.

The following antibodies are found in women with autoimmune disease. Their presence increases the risk of infertility and miscarriage. These antibodies increase the risk of blood clots which impair circulation to the fetus, thus the fetus can be lost through miscarriage. These antibodies can also inhibit implantation of the embryo in the uterine lining.

Cardiolipin antibodies

Cardiolipin is a component of the inner membrane of mitochondria inside your cells. Mitochondria are the structures that generate energy inside your cells. Cardiolipin antibodies are seen in patients with antiphospholipid syndrome and systemic lupus erthematosus, and other autoimmune diseases. The presence of cardiolipin antibodies may sometimes give a false positive reading in a syphilis test. Women with cardiolipin antibodies are more prone to blood clots, infertility and miscarriage.

Lupus inhibitor antibodies/lupus anticoagulant

These antibodies are associated with systemic lupus erythematosus, infertility and recurrent miscarriage.

Anti-sperm antibodies

A blood test can check whether a woman is making antibodies against her partner's sperm.

Other blood tests

Coagulation studies

Several blood tests are available to check for the presence of thrombophilia, meaning an excess tendency to form blood clots. Blood clots in and around the uterus and placenta can cause infertility or miscarriage.

Blood group and antibody test

Before falling pregnant you should have a test to check your blood type and Rh status. Approximately 15 percent of women lack the Rh factor on their red blood cells, therefore they are called Rh negative. Women who do have the factor on their red blood cells are called Rh positive. Rh refers to Rhesus, since it was first discovered in Rhesus monkeys. If an Rh negative woman is pregnant with an Rh positive baby, she can make antibodies against the baby's red blood cells, thereby causing fetal death. This problem can be prevented by giving a pregnant woman Rh immunoglobulin.

Tests for infections

Many infections produce extremely mild symptoms or no symptoms at all. However they can lead to infertility in women and men, or put your baby at risk if you do fall pregnant. The following tests may be required if you are having difficulty conceiving.

Chlamydia test

A urine test, blood test, cervical swab and urethral swab (in men) are all used to detect chlamydia. A high cervical swab is required when testing for genitourinary infections, as the infection may be hiding high up in the cervix and can be missed otherwise.

Gonorrhoea test

A urine test can detect the presence of gonorrhoea in women and men. Women should also have a high cervical swab performed, and men should have a swab taken from the urethra (opening at the tip of the penis).

Syphilis test

A blood test is done to check for the presence of antibodies to the organism that causes syphilis, called Treponema pallidum. Syphilis infection is rare, however if you do fall pregnant while infected, it is extremely harmful to the fetus. That is why your doctor will probably test you for this infection.

Rubella test

A blood test is done to check for levels of IgG rubella antibodies. This will determine if you have immunity to rubella. Contracting rubella while pregnant can cause birth defects in your baby; therefore you may wish to consider becoming vaccinated before attempting conception.

Cytomegalovirus test

A blood test is performed to check for the presence of antibodies to cytomegalovirus.

Toxoplasmosis test

Being infected with toxoplasmosis while pregnant would be dangerous for your developing baby. People become infected with toxoplasmosis through contact with cat feces or under cooked meat.

Additional investigations

The following tests may be required in the investigation of infertility.

Pelvic ultrasound (transvaginal ultrasound)

Having a pelvic ultrasound provides valuable information about the health of your uterus and ovaries, and can detect the presence of several abnormalities. These include fibroids, adenomyosis, ovarian endometriomas or other ovarian cysts. Adenomyosis refers to endometrial tissue (the lining of the uterus) within the myometrium (the thick, muscular layer of the uterus). Unfortunately a pelvic ultrasound cannot detect subtle abnormalities, and more specific tests may be required. It also does not provide any information about the health of your fallopian tubes. Sometimes an antral follicle count is performed during a pelvic ultrasound, in order to assess ovarian reserve. However, this method is much less accurate than a blood test for anti-mullerian hormone, and it must be conducted by an extremely experienced technician.

Hysterosalpingography

This is an X ray that shows the inside of your uterus and fallopian tubes. It can detect the presence of blockages or growths. It is most commonly done to check if the fallopian tubes are blocked. The test is performed during the first ten days of your menstrual cycle. A doctor injects a small amount of solution through your cervix into your uterus. This makes your uterus and fallopian tubes stretch.

An X ray machine is placed over your abdomen which takes pictures of your uterus and fallopian tubes. If your fallopian tubes are not blocked, the fluid will spill out of your tubes at the ends where your ovaries are. If your tubes are blocked, this will be seen on the X ray because the fluid will appear stuck inside. When the test is finished, the fluid is absorbed or it drains out of your vagina. You should not have a hysterosalpingogram if there is even the slightest chance that you are pregnant or if you are taking the drug metformin.

We do not recommend you have a hystrosalpingogram because the test uses radiation. You do not want X rays anywhere near your ovaries because your eggs contain the genetic material that you will pass on to your children. X rays cause DNA damage. That is the last thing you need. Instead, we recommend you have a similar test that uses an ultrasound instead of an X ray. It is called hysterosalpingo contrast sonography (HyCoSy).

Hysterosalpingo contrast sonography (HyCoSy)

This test uses an ultrasound instead of an X ray to check whether your fallopian tubes are blocked. It is a much safer test and we recommend you have it done instead of hysterosalpingography. A small amount of solution is injected into your uterus, to see whether there are any blockages in your fallopian tubes. Saline solution can be flushed through your tubes and this can open minor blockages, improving your chance of conception. This is a very specialized test, so we highly recommend you have it performed at an ultrasound practice that specializes in gynecological ultrasound.

Both the X ray and ultrasound techniques are usually quite uncomfortable, and even painful. The dye that gets injected through your cervix can cause painful uterine contractions, giving you period-like pain. Therefore your doctor will probably recommend you take a pain killer like aspirin or ibuprofen an hour before having the procedure.

Laparoscopy

This test may be required to check for the presence of endometriosis in women with very painful menstrual periods. It is also used in women who have had surgery to the reproductive tract in the past, to check for adhesions and other scar tissue, and to check for ovarian cysts. Sometimes laparoscopy is used to have a closer look at abnormalities detected by ultrasound. This procedure gives the most detailed information about the health of your reproductive organs but it is the most invasive test.

A laparoscopy is performed under general anaesthetic and allows a gynecologist to closely inspect your uterus, ovaries and fallopian tubes. A cut is made below your belly button. A needle is inserted through the cut and your abdomen gets inflated with carbon dioxide gas. A laparoscope (type of telescope) is then inserted into the cut in your abdomen, which gives your doctor a very clear image of your pelvic organs. A sample of tissue may be taken from your pelvis, for examination by a pathologist. Small growths and scar tissue can be removed using this procedure.

Hysteroscopy

A diagnostic hysteroscopy typically only takes a few minutes, and can be done while you are awake. A hysteroscope (similar to a narrow telescope) is inserted through the cervix into the uterus in order to obtain a clear view of the uterine lining. Typically, a sample of endometrial tissue is taken during the procedure, to be analyzed by a pathologist. A hysteroscopy is sometimes performed to remove small uterine fibroids, uterine polyps, or to cut intra uterine adhesions.

Hair Mineral Analysis

This is an extremely useful test to check for heavy metal toxicity. Blood tests are not a reliable way to check for heavy metals because they do not tend to stay in your bloodstream for long. Heavy metals tend to get stored in our organs and bones. Blood tests are most useful to check for acute heavy metal toxicity. In most cases it is chronic exposure to heavy metals that builds up over time and leads to health problems, including infertility. Being deficient in essential minerals makes you more prone to heavy metal toxicity.

Your naturopath or doctor can arrange for a sample of your hair to be sent to a laboratory for analysis. In order to check for recent heavy metal toxicity, it is important to cut a sample of hair as close to the roots as possible. You will need to provide approximately two tablespoons of hair for analysis. Recent improvements in testing methods have meant that it doesn't matter if your hair is dyed; it can still be accurately tested.

11. Male infertility

For many years it was thought that if a couple were having difficulties conceiving, it must be because of problems with the woman. We now know that male factor infertility is extremely common and indeed male factors are currently responsible for 40 percent of infertility. Around ten percent of men in the USA are considered infertile. Approximately one in 20 Australian men is now considered infertile![115]

Luckily, in the majority of cases male infertility is easier and faster to remedy than female infertility. Most cases of infertility are caused by problems with sperm manufacture. Sperm are incredibly sensitive to a man's diet and environment, and we will show you how to modify those in order to boost the production of healthy sperm. A man's health is just as important as a woman's health when preparing to conceive a child, as 50 percent of the DNA that makes up the child is contributed by the sperm.

Infertility may affect more men than women!

This is according to figures released at the 21st annual conference of the European Society of Human Reproduction and Embryology. A report that monitors assisted reproduction in Europe, has shown that ICSI (intracytoplasmic sperm injection) overtook conventional IVF techniques as the most commonly used assisted reproductive technology in Europe in 2002. According to figures released from 24 European countries in 2002, there were more than 122, 000 ICSI cycles and nearly 113, 000 IVF cycles. ICSI is used when sperm quality is sub-optimal. If the sperm is not able to penetrate the egg when left to its own devices, it is injected into an egg by a fertility doctor[116]

The male reproductive system

Before we explain sperm production, we will give you a basic overview of the male reproductive system, so you can see where potential problems may originate.

Male reproductive organs

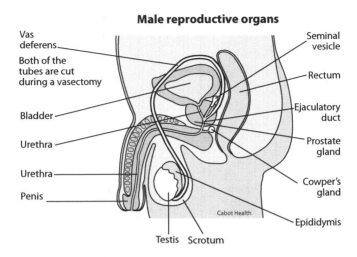

The most important reproductive organs in men are the testes, as they produce sperm and also produce the hormone testosterone. The testes hang in the scrotal sac. They need to be outside the body, as sperm production requires a temperature two to three degrees lower than body temperature. Sperm are transported away from each testicle by a long tube called the epididymis. These tubes have many coils in them and while they are in the epididymis, sperm cells mature and gain the ability to swim. The journey along the epididymis takes approximately 20 days.

A tube called the vas deferens joins the epididymis and transports sperm to the prostate gland. The vas deferens is the tube that is cut when men undergo a vasectomy. The vas deferens empties into the ejaculatory duct, which passes through the prostate gland and joins with the urethra. The urethra is the tube through which semen is ejaculated out of the body, and also the tube that carries urine from the bladder and out of the body. The prostate is a walnut shaped gland that sits below the bladder. The prostate and the seminal vesicles produce fluids that make up the semen, and nourish the sperm. Each ejaculate consists of a thick mixture of sugars, citric acid, vitamins, minerals and other ingredients to provide the sperm with energy for the massive journey ahead. Sperm make up only approximately one percent of the semen mass.

Sperm production

Sperm production takes between 74 and 78 days.[117] The process is called spermatogenesis. Women are already born with all the eggs they will ever have inside their ovaries, and they rapidly deteriorate as a woman ages. In men, sperm production begins at puberty and doesn't stop until a man dies. A young and healthy man produces more than four million new sperm per hour in each testicle! The quantity of sperm produced does diminish greatly with age and the quality of the sperm also deteriorates. Men are born with the immature cells that will eventually be converted into sperm in their testes (called germ cells). The other major cells found inside the testes are called Sertoli cells and Leydig cells. Sertoli cells nourish the developing sperm and produce hormones. Leydig cells produce testosterone.

Sperm are one of the tiniest cells of the human body. The head of a mature sperm cell spans across only two-thousandths of an inch. This is less than half the width of a white blood cell or skin cell. In contract, the female egg is one of the biggest cells of the human body; it is 30 times the width of a sperm cell and is big enough to be seen with the naked eye.

Structure of the sperm

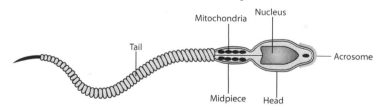

Sperm are made of three important sections, a head, midpiece and a tail. The head contains 23 tightly packed chromosomes (the genes), which hope to combine with the 23 chromosomes inside the female egg to form one cell. The tip of the head contains the acrosome, which is a sack containing specialized enzymes that help the sperm to penetrate through the female reproductive tract and eventually the waiting egg. Below the head is the midpiece. This section is packed with tiny structures called mitochondria. Mitochondria are rod shaped tiny organs that generate energy inside cells. Muscle cells, heart cells and sperm cells all contain high numbers of mitochondria because they are all hard working cells with very high energy requirements. Unfortunately mitochondria are extremely sensitive structures and they are easily destroyed or compromised by environmental chemicals, free radicals and unhealthy lifestyles. Low quantity or poor quality mitochondria inside sperm cells affect sperm motility; that is the ability of sperm to swim.

The third part of the sperm is the tail. It comprises a bundle of 11 entwined filaments that thrash and propel the sperm forward. Because sperm cells take approximately three months to form, all men who wish to have children must clean up their diet and strive to achieve optimum health for at least three months before trying to conceive.

What causes male infertility?

The following factors are responsible for the majority of male infertility:

Sperm problems

Low sperm count, motility problems (ability to swim) and morphology problems (abnormal shape) are the most common cause of male infertility. Therefore the first step when investigating a male for infertility is to perform a semen analysis. This gives us a great deal of information about what the sperm look and behave like, and it can give us information about the quality of DNA inside the sperm. Many factors affect sperm production and quality and they are covered in detail later in this chapter.

Structural problems

The next most common cause of male infertility is obstruction of the tubes that carry sperm from the testes to the penis. This may be caused by previous sexually transmitted infection that was not treated promptly or adequately. Obstruction of the tubes can cause a complete lack of sperm in the semen. Men who have had a vasectomy, and then attempted to have it reversed can also fall into this category.

Infertility is more common in men who had undescended testes in infancy, and required surgery to correct this. The presence of hypospadias at birth is also a risk factor. Hypospadias is a condition whereby the urethra does not open at the tip of the penis. Instead the opening is found along the underside of the penis, or even in the perineum. Surgery is used to correct this. Both undescended testes and hypospadias are associated with chemical exposure while a man was a fetus inside his mother's uterus.

Hormonal problems

Hormonal factors are uncommon and affect less than one in 100 infertile men. Sometimes the pituitary gland in the brain does not produce adequate levels of hormones that control the testes' production of testosterone and sperm. The use of anabolic, androgenic steroids by body builders can shut off hormone production by the pituitary gland and lead to a low sperm count. Thyroid disorders in males affect fertility. Excess prolactin produced by the pituitary gland can lead to infertility

Sexual problems

Erectile dysfunction can cause fertility problems because it impairs the delivery of sperm to the female reproductive tract. In the vast majority of cases, erectile dysfunction is a symptom of poor health and specifically poor cardiovascular health. The arteries of the penis are much more narrow than arteries that travel to the heart or brain, therefore they tend to get blocked with cholesterol first. Erectile dysfunction is often an early warning sign of an impending heart attack or stroke. Weight loss, regular exercise and a healthy diet will remedy this problem in the majority of cases. Some medication to treat depression or high blood pressure can cause erection problems. Some men with diabetes suffer a condition known as retrograde ejaculation. This is where instead of spurting out of the penis, semen spills upwards and into the bladder instead. Spinal cord injuries can also be responsible for ejaculation difficulties.

Immune system disorders

Some women produce antibodies against their partner's sperm, but men can produce antibodies against their own sperm as well. The antibodies bind to the sperm and inactivate them. The antibodies can be detected in semen and in the bloodstream.

The semen analysis

This is the first step in determining whether a male is infertile, and this test should be carried out in all couples who have not been successful at conception for a year or more. The test results will be most accurate if the semen is analyzed not more than an hour after ejaculation. It is also important for a man to abstain from ejaculation for more than two days, but less than seven days before having this test. Normal semen parameters are listed below:

World Health Organization Reference Values for Semen Analysis Testing

Volume .... *> 2mL*

Sperm concentration .... *> 20 million/mL*

Sperm number .... *> 40 million per ejaculate*

Sperm motility .... *> 50% progressive or > 25% rapidly progressive*

Morphology .... *> 15% normal forms*

White blood cells .... *< 1 million/mL*

Immunobead or mixed antiglobulin reaction test .... *< 10% coated*

Vitality .... *greater than or equal to 75% living*

pH .... *greater than or equal to 7.2*

Liquefaction time .... *< 60 minutes*

When having a semen analysis performed, we strongly recommend you also request a test for sperm antibodies and a test called a sperm chromatin structure assay. This is explained in the section that follows. A man should not have a semen analysis performed if he has had a fever in the previous three months, as raised body temperature impairs sperm production.

How to interpret a semen analysis

The report that accompanies the test results will contain terms you are probably not familiar with. Some terms are self explanatory; the rest are explained below:

- **Sperm concentration and number:** When providing a semen sample, it is very important to make sure you collect all of the semen. The semen released first contains the highest number of sperm, and the semen released last contains far fewer sperm. Not providing the entire semen sample can give a false reading; either very high sperm count or very low sperm count.
- **Sperm motility:** This measures the ability of sperm to move. Sperm are classified as either: rapidly progressive, slowly progressive, non-progressive or immotile.
- **Sperm morphology:** This test analyzes the shape of the sperm. It checks for the presence of a normal head, mid-piece and tail. Sperm with abnormal morphology are not able to penetrate the egg, and if they do, the pregnancy typically results in miscarriage.
- **pH test:** Semen should be highly alkaline. Acidic sperm is an indicator of poor systemic health and high levels of inflammation in the body, or infection.
- **White blood cells:** High numbers of white blood cells indicate an active infection. Genitourinary infections can affect sperm production, sperm quality and can block the tubes that carry the sperm to the penis.
- **Liquefaction time:** Immediately after ejaculation, semen is a thick mucus-like consistency. Normal semen changes to a watery liquid within 15 to 60 minutes.

Based on the results of the semen analysis, a man will be given a sperm classification using the following terminology:

- **Normozoospermia:** This indicates the sperm in the semen are normal enough to meet the World Health Organization criteria.
- **Oligozoospermia:** This refers to semen in which the sperm concentration is too low; below the World Health Organization reference value. Between 5 and 20 million sperm per milliliter classifies as mild to moderate oligozoospermia, while a level less than five million classifies as severe oligozoospermia. The various causes of low sperm count are listed in the section that follows.
- **Asthenozoospermia:** This refers to a high number of sperm with poor motility.

- **Teratozoospermia:** Refers to a large number of sperm with abnormal morphology.
- **Oligoasthenoteratozoospermia:** This describes the condition when all sperm variables are below the normal levels set by the World Health Organization.
- **Azoospermia:** A condition where no sperm at all are present in the semen.
- **Leucocytospermia:** Refers to high levels of white blood cells in the semen.
- **Necrozoospermia:** All of the sperm in the semen are non-viable or non-motile.

In most cases there is more than one problem with the sperm; low sperm count usually goes hand in hand with poor motility and poor morphology. It only takes one sperm to fertilize an egg, therefore a sperm count of less than 20 million per milliliter sounds like there are still plenty of sperm to do the job. However, the factors that cause low sperm numbers almost always cause poor sperm quality as well.

Testing the DNA inside sperm

A standard semen analysis is an extremely useful test but it does not give us information about the quality of the DNA inside sperm. There is another test you should request called the Sperm Chromatin Structure Assay (SCSA). This test tells us what percentage of sperm has abnormal DNA. Sperm quality is dependent on the amount of damage present in sperm DNA; also known as DNA fragmentation. The DNA inside our cells is arranged in a double helix, or ladder configuration, with side rails and rungs. If the rungs are broken, the ladder becomes unsteady and cannot function properly. Recent studies have shown that we cannot predict how much DNA fragmentation (damage) is present in sperm just by the way they look. A standard semen analysis will not reveal this information. Men with normal sperm counts, normal sperm morphology and motility can still have high levels of DNA fragmentation. The more DNA damage is present inside the sperm, the more difficulties a couple will experience when trying to conceive.

The test used to determine the degree of DNA fragmentation inside sperm is called the Sperm Chromatin Structure Assay. The genetic material contained inside the head of the sperm is called chromatin. This test measures the integrity of the chromatin. A computerised test measures the percentage of damaged sperm, giving an index known as the DNA Fragmentation Index (DFI). A normal sperm sample contains less than 15 percent of sperm with DNA damage. Men with poor fertility have more than 30 percent of their sperm with DNA damage.

A DNA Fragmentation Index greater than 30 percent is associated with:

* A longer time period to establish a normal pregnancy
* Increased incidence of miscarriage
* Failure to achieve pregnancy[118]

Normally, sperm that contain high levels of DNA fragmentation would not be able to initiate conception, or a full term pregnancy. However, with assisted reproductive technologies, particularly ICSI, these sperm are able to achieve conception and pregnancy. Enabling sperm with genetic damage to achieve pregnancy may lead to an increased incidence of genetic diseases and childhood cancer in the offspring.[119] Children born from these sperm are at increased risk of low birth weight, congenital abnormalities including neural tube defects and hypospadias, as well as an increased risk of visual, cardiac and neurological impairments.[120] Assisted reproductive technologies (ART) are implicated as a major risk factor for some childhood cancers. For example, children born through ART have a six fold higher risk of retinoblastoma.[121] Retinoblastoma is a rapidly developing cancer of the retina in the eyes. For this reason, some researchers speculate that it may take several generations before the full consequences of using DNA damaged sperm in ART such as IVF are realized![122]

For these reasons, it is vital that all couples planning to use assisted reproductive technologies have a sperm chromatin structure assay performed on the sperm to check the level of DNA damage present. This is vitally important to protect the future health of your child.

How does the DNA inside sperm get damaged?

Damage to DNA in any cell in the body (not just sperm calls) is mostly caused by free radical damage. Men with high levels of DNA fragmentation have high levels of free radicals in their semen. Free radical damage is caused by radiation, exposure to environmental chemicals, poor diet, lack of antioxidants in the diet and nutrient deficiencies. The combination of chemical exposure and nutrient deficiencies causes the greatest harm. If you have high levels of vitamins, minerals and essential fatty acids in your diet, they will offer you a great deal of protection against harmful substances in the environment.

It is very interesting to consider that DNA damage inside sperm cells is an indicator of DNA damage inside other cells of your body too. Older men (older than 40) have higher levels of DNA fragmentation inside sperm. As all of us get older, mistakes occur more commonly in our DNA as our cells replicate.
Also the older we are, the longer we have been exposed to environmental chemicals. These chemicals accumulate inside our bodies and we are said to have a greater "body burden" of chemicals.

Therefore men with high levels of DNA fragmentation inside their sperm cells can usually consider themselves at higher risk of cancer. This is not always the case, because sometimes simple factors such as heat or a varicocele may be responsible for the raised level of DNA damage. Luckily the DNA fragmentation index can be improved with diet and lifestyle changes, as well as the use of specific nutrients. The factors that cause low sperm counts and high levels of abnormal sperm are often also responsible for DNA damage inside sperm.

The rapid worldwide decline in sperm counts

Sperm counts have been falling dramatically in the last 60 years, and if they continue at the same pace we may end up with more infertile men than fertile men. According to the World Health Organization, a normal sperm count is more than 20 million sperm per milliliter of semen. It is interesting to note that the so-called normal reference values have been falling in recent years; they have had to, otherwise very few normal men would be able to satisfy these criteria. Not only are sperm counts falling; levels of sperm with abnormal shape or movement are increasing.

Professor Niels Skakkeback was a Danish scientist who first alerted the world to the possibility of a substantial fall in male fertility levels in 1992. He demonstrated that sperm counts in healthy men had dropped by more than half in 50 years. Professor Skakkeback and his team, in the Department of Growth and Development at Copenhagen University reviewed 61 international studies involving 14,947 men between 1938 and 1992.[123] They found that the average sperm count had fallen from 113 million per milliliter in 1940 to 66 million in 1990. Even worse, the definition of a "normal" sperm count fell from 60 million per milliliter to 20 million in the same period.

Other researchers have found a similar trend. A survey of 1,350 sperm donors in Paris found a decline in sperm counts by approximately two percent each year over the past 23 years. Interestingly younger men had the poorest quality semen.[124] In another study conducted at the University of Helsinki, testicular tissue was examined at post-mortem from 528 middle aged Finnish men who died suddenly in either 1981 or 1991.[125] Of the men who died in 1981, 56.4 percent had normal, healthy sperm production. By 1991, only 26.9 percent of men were producing healthy sperm.

Currently, according to the World Health Organization, a man is classified as normal if more than 15 percent of the sperm he produces are normal. That means it is now considered "normal" to manufacture almost 85 percent abnormal sperm! That's outrageous! According to Dr Harry Fisch, a urologist at Columbia Medical Center in the USA, "a man is lucky if 15 percent of his sperm are serviceable. One guy I saw had 22 percent, but that's rare". These statistics are absolutely frightening. Luckily new sperm are produced every three months, and changes in a man's diet and lifestyle produce dramatic improvements in the quality and quantity of his sperm.

Why is sperm quality and quantity falling so dramatically?

Often, men with an abnormal semen analysis result are told their problem is genetic. We disagree. Such dramatic drops in sperm counts cannot be explained by genetic factors; lifestyle and environmental factors must be to blame and there is a large body of research to support this. It is thought that endocrine disruptors are having the greatest impact on male reproductive health. Endocrine disruptors are also known as xeno-estrogens (false estrogens).

The ability of men to manufacture sperm is limited by two factors: the efficiency of the process of sperm production (spermatogenesis) and the number of Sertoli cells (supportive cells) present in the testes. The cells of the testes are formed while a man is inside his mother's uterus. Therefore the health of his mother and the chemicals she was exposed to while pregnant with him have an enormous bearing on a man's future potential to manufacture sperm. When a man's mother is exposed to a higher level of endocrine disruptors while pregnant, the man is born with fewer Sertoli cells inside his testes. This restricts the amount of sperm he can manufacture for the rest of his life

Leading UK scientist Professor Richard Sharpe, of the Medical Research Council believes that many chemicals in consumer products such as cosmetics and cleaning products are partly responsible for infertility in men and birth defects in children. Low sperm counts, malformations of the penis (hypospadias), undescended testes and testicular cancer are all becoming increasingly common in recent decades. This is referred to as "testicular dysgenesis syndrome". Dysgenesis means abnormal development of an organ.

The origin of these problems can be traced back to development in the uterus. In a male fetus, testosterone is required in high amounts in order to form a normal penis and make the testicles descend. Professor Sharpe and many other researchers believe that many commonly used chemicals block the action of testosterone in the uterus, and therefore harm the future reproductive health of the child. Professor Sharpe also believes that these various chemicals are not so much a threat on their own, but become a bigger problem when they are all mixed together. Unfortunately no one researches the effects of combined exposure to chemicals on our health and probably never will. Industry and the economy depend very heavily on these harmful chemicals and it is not in the interest of the government to investigate their true effects on human health. Minimizing your exposure to environmental chemicals will not only help you to achieve conception in the near future, it will help to protect the fertility of your children and your children's children.

What causes low sperm count?

The following list describes the most common factors that reduce sperm count, as well as reduce sperm quality:

Varicoceles

Varicoceles are dilated veins in the testes. The veins in the testes, (just like the veins in the legs) contain valves that help blood to move upward towards the heart. If the valves stop working, blood pools in the veins and they bulge.

Varicoceles are very common; approximately 15 percent of men have them. However they are often mild and cause no symptoms or problems. Sometimes varicoceles are a significant problem, and in fact 40 percent of infertile men have a varicocele.[126] Varicoceles usually cause low sperm count, poor morphology and low motility. They affect the left testicle more often because of the architecture of the veins on that side. The pooling of blood that varicoceles cause, raises the temperature in the testes. This greatly reduces a man's ability to produce sperm and the heat triggers sperm abnormalities.

In most cases varicocele can be diagnosed via a physical examination and ultrasound. A large varicocele can make the scrotum look lumpy, so it resembles a bag of worms. Surgery can successfully repair a varicocele, and a repeat semen analysis should be performed four months later. In most cases sperm concentrations return to normal. Men with varicoceles need to increase their intake of nutrients that improve the structural integrity of veins; these include vitamin C, bioflavonoids, the herbs horse chestnut (Aesculus hippocastanum) and butcher's broom (Ruscus aculeatus).

Heat

Excess heat around the testes greatly impairs sperm production. The testes require a temperature two to three degrees lower than body temperature in order to manufacture sperm. Factors that increase testicular heat include the use of hot spas and saunas, tight underpants, being overweight and resting a laptop computer on your lap. Put it on a table instead. A fever raises testicular temperature. If a man has had a fever, he should wait three months before having a semen analysis, as this would greatly affect the outcome.

Immune system disorders

Some men produce antibodies against their own sperm. Risk factors for this include testicular trauma, previous genitourinary infection, history of testicular surgery and previous large varicocele. Sperm antibody production is also higher in men with autoimmune disease, allergies and nutritional deficiencies; particularly deficiencies in vitamin D, selenium and zinc.

Men with sperm antibodies must follow the anti-inflammatory guidelines in chapter 5. Conventional medicine uses steroids for the treatment of this condition. Steroids have terrible side effects and they are usually not required because nutritional medicine offers so many potent anti-inflammatory agents.

Medication

Several prescription medications affect the sperm count. They include:

- Ketoconazole (an anti-fungal)
- Sulfasalazine (used for inflammatory bowel disease)
- Cimetidine (for reflux or ulcers)
- Blood pressure drugs that are calcium channel blockers. Examples include Norvasc and Adalat.
- Spironolactone (a diuretic)
- Some antibiotics: erythromycin, gentamicin and nitrofuran
- Cholesterol lowering drugs
- Some antidepressants
- Steroids

Selective Serotonin Reuptake Inhibitors (SSRIs) are some of the most widely prescribed antidepressants. Studies have shown that these drugs increase the amount of DNA fragmentation inside sperm; typically to 30 percent or greater. This is a level high enough to classify a man as infertile. All men taking SSRI medication should have a sperm chromatin structure assay test to check if the health of their sperm is being affected. Sperm DNA typically returns to normal within a month or two of discontinuing the medication.

Steroids can interfere with the proper development of sperm. Cortisone injections (such as for joint pain) can cause a DNA fragmentation index in sperm cells well above 30 percent. This effect wears off a month or so after the injection. Lower levels of cortisone are commonly prescribed for immune system conditions and still affect sperm health, but less dramatically. Cholesterol lowering drugs can increase DNA fragmentation in sperm more than 40 percent.

Complete lack of sperm (azoospermia)

This is a rare scenario where there are virtually no sperm present in the semen. This can be caused by a failure in sperm production, or a blockage somewhere that is preventing sperm from travelling to the penis. The three main causes of lack of sperm production are: hormonal problems, testicular failure and varicocele. Hormones made by the hypothalamus and pituitary gland in the brain stimulate the production of sperm in the testes. If inadequate levels of these hormones are produced, sperm production is compromised. Men who take anabolic steroids (for example body builders) shut down the production of hormones required for sperm formation.

Testicular failure refers to an inability of the sperm-producing part of the testicle to produce adequate quantities of mature sperm. Sometimes the testicles completely lack the cells that divide to become sperm (this is called Sertoli cell-only syndrome). In other instances the sperm are unable to complete the maturation process (called maturation arrest). Genetic abnormalities are the most common cause of these conditions.

Blockages of the epididymis or vas deferens can prevent sperm from travelling from the testes to the penis. These blockages are usually caused by infections, or damage incurred by previous surgery for varicocele or an inguinal hernia. Occasionally one or more tubes are absent because of a congenital abnormality (the men were born that way). Sperm are stored in sacs called the seminal vesicles, and are then deposited in the urethra, which is the tube through which men urinate and ejaculate. The sperm must pass through the ejaculatory ducts to get from the seminal vesicles to the urethra. If these are blocked on both sides, the sperm will not be able to come through. Surgery may be used to correct such blockages. If the blockages can't be corrected, surgery can still be used to retrieve sperm from the testes, where they can be used in IVF, ICSI or intrauterine insemination.

Hormonal disorders

Men with an over active thyroid gland experience impaired sperm production and impaired sperm motility. Premature ejaculation is sometimes a feature of hyperthyroidism. These abnormalities are improved once thyroid hormone production is corrected. Loss of libido and erectile dysfunction may be present with an over active or under active thyroid gland.[127, 128]

Excess production of the hormone prolactin inhibits the production of testosterone and sperm. Along with causing infertility, high prolactin levels can also cause a loss of sex drive and erectile dysfunction. Excess prolactin production is usually caused by a small tumor in the brain which over secretes prolactin. Medication is available for this condition.

Ageing

A great deal of research has shown that sperm DNA fragmentation increases with age. All men over 40 years of age must have a sperm chromatin structure assay test. A study analyzing 17,000 cycles of intrauterine insemination (IUI) showed that the pregnancy rate was 14.4 percent among men younger than 30 years, and dropped to 8.9 percent among men older than 42 years. The increased incidence of DNA fragmentation inside sperm is thought to be responsible.

Diet and lifestyle factors

A great number of lifestyle factors impair sperm production and reduce sperm quality. These are some of the leading causes of male infertility. Thankfully, improvements in diet and lifestyle usually have dramatic effects in improving sperm quality. Men who are overweight or obese often have fertility problems.

Obesity in men is associated with lower testosterone, higher estrogen, lower sperm count and poor semen quality.[129] Fat cells in obese men convert much of the testosterone in their body into estrogen. Obese men also have poor outcomes with IVF and other assisted reproductive technologies.

A University of Adelaide, Australia study of couples undergoing IVF found that as paternal Body Mass Index (BMI) increased, clinical pregnancy rates were significantly reduced.

Pregnancy was achieved in almost half of the couples where the male was a normal weight, but in only a quarter of couples where the male was overweight or obese. Where the male was morbidly obese, less than ten percent of couples achieved pregnancy. The authors of the study state that obesity may be linked to DNA damage and oxidative stress (inflammation), which have a negative impact on male fertility.[130] The fat cells in your body produce a host of inflammatory chemicals that cause wear and tear to your body and damage to the DNA inside your cells. Obese men also have a higher testicular body temperature, as fat from the abdomen hangs down towards the testicles.

Nutritional deficiencies

Deficiencies in vitamins, minerals, essential fatty acids and antioxidants can have terrible effects on sperm health. The most important nutrients for male fertility are listed on page 217.

Radiation

Radiation has a very detrimental effect on sperm production. Modern life means we are bombarded with numerous sources of radiation; many of these cannot be avoided, but some can. Research has linked mobile phone use to reduced sperm quality. Men who carry mobile phones in their pocket, or clipped to their belt expose their testes to an amount of radiation significant enough to cause a reduction in sperm motility and viability. The semen of these men contains higher amounts of reactive oxygen species, which basically means higher amounts of free radical damage.[131]

The damage is greatest when the phone is clipped to the waist and in talk mode while using a bluetooth device. If you use bluetooth, do not keep the phone against your body. Clip it somewhere in the car, put it on a bench or hold it in your hand. When appropriate, it is also advisable to use the speakerphone option while talking on your mobile phone. As long as the phone is not attached to your body at the time.

Electric blankets are another obvious source of electromagnetic radiation that can easily be avoided, and men should not rest laptop computers on their laps. Radiation is well known to cause damage to the DNA inside our cells.

Chemicals

Chemicals are very capable of having adverse effects on sperm production. In today's world we are all exposed to an ever increasing array of chemicals, and it is impossible to avoid them entirely. Numerous studies have linked increasing levels of air pollution to declining sperm quality. All men are exposed to most of the chemicals that are described in this section, however men in certain occupations are more prone to infertility; these occupations include: rubber, petroleum and agricultural chemical workers; painters, mechanics, welders and cleaners.

A great deal of research has been published in the brilliant journal Environmental Health Perspectives, linking paternal exposure to various chemicals with miscarriage, low birth weight, birth defects, genital defects in male offspring, childhood leukemia and brain cancer, as well as a change in the male to female sex ratio of offspring. More males have always been born than females. Worldwide, around 106 boys are born for every 100 girls. The fact is that fewer boys make it to adulthood, so this is probably Mother Nature's way of balancing the numbers. In recent years this ratio is changing and males exposed to greater levels of chemicals, especially dioxins, are more likely to father girls.

Why are the testes so susceptible to environmental chemicals?

Unlike the ovaries, the testes are home to extremely rapidly dividing cells. Millions of sperm are produced each day. Rapidly dividing cells anywhere in the body are more prone to mistakes in DNA replication. The precursor cells that eventually become sperm are also involved in extremely complex cell differentiation (specialization). As sperm cells mature and take on their characteristic shape of a head, midpiece and tail, the steps involved in that process are extremely sensitive to chemical exposure. Therefore, rapid cell division and specialization make sperm cells highly sensitive to environmental chemicals.

The eggs in a woman's ovaries are all present before a woman is even born; with each menstrual cycle several eggs ripen and mature. That process in females is far less susceptible to harm caused by chemicals. So we can say that men must be just as careful to avoid environmental chemicals and drugs before conception as women need to be while pregnant!

Chemicals that have been shown to impair sperm quality and/or quantity:

Pesticides: DDT is one of the most studied pesticides in relation to its effects on fertility. DDT was the first widely used synthetic pesticide, and although it has been banned in most countries, it is still present in the environment. DDT takes an incredibly long time to break down; therefore small amounts are found in the body fat and breast milk of just about every person on the planet today. Organophosphate pesticides are known to increase DNA fragmentation in sperm cells. Men employed in agriculture receive the highest exposure, however these pesticides are widely used on a range of food crops today and it is impossible not to ingest some of these pesticides.

Phthalates: Pronounced "thal ates", these are chemicals that improve flexibility in a range of plastic products. Phthalates are also widely found in personal care products, flooring, adhesives and cologne. They are usually a component of fragrance in personal care products. Research has shown that higher urine levels of phthalates correspond with higher levels of DNA damage in sperm.[132]

Bisphenol A: This is a building block of polycarbonate plastic. It is used in some plastic water bottles, as well as the inner white lining of some canned foods, epoxy resins and dental sealants. Experiments in mice have shown that bisphenol A significantly reduces sperm production in a dose dependent manner. An acceptable daily intake of bisphenol A in the USA is considered to be up to 50 micrograms per kilogram of body weight. Experiments done on mice have shown adverse effects on sperm production at a dose of 20 micrograms per kilogram.[133]

Personal lubricants: Be careful which lubricant you use, as most of them contain substances that have been shown to damage sperm. Most commercial lubricants reduce the ability of sperm to swim, reduce their viability, and even cause DNA damage inside sperm cells. A study published in the *International Journal of Fertility and Menopausal Studies* examined the effects of four commercially available personal lubricants (Touch, Astroglide, Replens, and K-Y Jelly) and two vegetable oil products (containing canola oil) on sperm motility and viability. Researchers took samples of sperm and mixed them with the lubricants. The effects on the sperm were measured at one, 15, 30, and 60 minute marks. All four commercial lubricants inhibited sperm motility by 60 to 100 percent after 60 minutes.[134]

It is very interesting to realize that the most commonly used spermicide, nonoxynol-9, which is present in spermicidal jells and foams is just as effective at killing sperm! In this particular study, canola oil had no effect on sperm, but we do not recommend it be used as a lubricant or consumed. There are natural personal lubricants available in health food stores and supermarkets that are less likely to cause harm to sperm, but they may still impair sperm motility because the lubricants change the pH of the vagina.

Heavy metals: Exposure to high levels of lead, cadmium and mercury can reduce sperm quality and quantity. See page 176 for information on reducing your exposure to these metals.

Additional tests in the investigation of male infertility

A semen analysis is usually the first and most important test done in the investigation of male infertility. If the result is abnormal, it should be repeated six weeks later. After implementing our diet and lifestyle recommendations, the test should be repeated three months later. Apart from a semen analysis, several other tests may need to be performed.

Blood tests should be performed for the following hormones:

Testosterone

The normal range of total testosterone in men is 8 – 27 nmol/L (230 - 778 ng/dL). The normal range for free testosterone is 170 – 510 pmol/L. Testosterone levels are often normal, even in men with significant sperm production problems.

Luteinizing hormone (LH)

In men LH stimulates testosterone production. The normal range is 2 – 10 U/L. If LH is high and testosterone is low, there is a problem with the testicular production of testosterone.

If both testosterone and LH are low, there may be a problem with the hypothalamus or pituitary gland in the brain. Sometimes this is caused by a prolactinoma (prolactin secreting tumor). In that case a prolactin blood test should be performed.

Follicle Stimulating hormone (FSH)

In men FSH stimulates sperm production. The normal range is 1.0 – 5.0 U/L. An elevated FSH level usually indicates a problem with sperm production in the testes (primary testicular failure).

Genetic testing

If the problem is recurrent miscarriage, the male will need a blood test to check for genetic problems, called karyotyping. This test involves counting the number of chromosomes in cells and checking for structural abnormalities in the chromosomes.

Along with blood tests, a man may need referral to a urologist who will perform a physical examination and ultrasound scans of the testes.

Infertile men at higher risk of testicular cancer and prostate cancer

Research has shown there is an association between male infertility and testicular cancer. This is especially so if a male was born with undescended testes. It is thought that exposure to endocrine disruptors while in his mother's uterus is responsible for these conditions. Testicular cancer usually occurs in young men; it is most common between the ages of 18 and 39. It usually begins as a painless lump in a testicle. All men should perform a testicular self exam regularly, and this is particularly important in men with a history of infertility. You can find instructions for a testicular self exam on this website: www. andrologyaustralia.org

Recent research has shown that men with a history of infertility are at greater risk of aggressive prostate cancer later in life.

Researchers from the University of Washington in Seattle tracked 22,500 men who attended one of 15 infertility clinics between 1967 and 1998. The researchers discovered that infertility increased the risk of being diagnosed with a slow growing prostate tumor 1.6 times, and aggressive tumors 2.6 times. The researchers speculated that this increased risk may be due to environmental toxin exposure while in the uterus, which caused damage to the male chromosome. Therefore men with a history of infertility may require more monitoring for prostate cancer, beginning around age 45.

Clearly it is too late to undo the harm caused by environmental chemicals while you or your partner were in your mother's uterus. However, this is a good reminder of why it is so important to limit your exposure to environmental chemicals before and during pregnancy, to reduce the risk of health problems later in your children's lives.

How to improve male fertility

The following recommendations must be adhered to for at least three months before attempting conception. While sperm cells are developing, they are incredibly sensitive to the effects of environmental chemicals, poor diet, radiation and nutrient deficiencies. The sperm contributes fifty percent of the DNA that makes up your baby; therefore the male has an enormous responsibility to bring his health to the highest possible level before conception is attempted.

Diet: All men should follow our diet recommendations described in chapter 8. Protein, good fats, vegetables and pure water are the basis of a healthy diet. Gluten and dairy products should be avoided in men who have anti-sperm antibodies, men who have an autoimmune disease and men who have symptoms of allergies described on page 82.

Antioxidants: Modern living has meant that our bodies are continually bombarded with chemicals that cause free radical damage, or oxidative damage to our cells. Stress, radiation exposure and nutrient deficiencies are all responsible. Sperm are highly susceptible to oxidative damage. Markers of oxidative damage can be measured in the semen and a great deal of research has shown that high degrees of oxidative damage correlate with impaired fertility. Free radical damage to sperm cells can damage the sperm cell membrane, reducing the ability of sperm to swim, and impairing their ability to penetrate an egg. It also damages the DNA inside sperm cells, thereby passing on defective DNA to the fetus. This increases the risk of infertility, miscarriage, congenital abnormalities, Down syndrome and other genetic disorders.

The following foods are an excellent source of antioxidants: vegetables, fruit, herbs and spices, nuts, seeds, green tea and dark chocolate. Try to include fresh herbs in your salads and cooking. Herbs are very easy to grow and they take up very little room; therefore you can grow a nice selection in pots or in a vegetable patch at home. Some examples of herbs you can grow at home include parsley, coriander, rocket, dill, basil, oregano, rosemary, chives and sage. Powdered spices are also potent antioxidants; some examples include turmeric, ground cumin, ground coriander root and paprika.

Nutritional supplements

The following nutritional supplements all greatly help to improve the quality and quantity of sperm. You will not be able to obtain sufficient levels of these nutrients through your diet.

Selenium: This mineral is the most important nutrient for male fertility. Selenium protects the DNA inside cells from damage; therefore it protects the DNA inside sperm from fragmentation.[135] Research has shown that selenium improves the health of Leydig cells inside testes, which are the cells that manufacture testosterone. This has the beneficial effect of improving sperm quality.[136] Selenium also helps to reduce the risk of miscarriage.[137] An optimal level of selenium supplementation is 200 micrograms per day.

Vitamin D: Australian research has shown that vitamin D deficiency compromises the health of sperm. Men who are deficient in this vitamin have more abnormal shaped sperm, and higher rates of DNA fragmentation inside their sperm. Men with anti-sperm antibodies are usually deficient in vitamin D. Vitamin D deficiency is extremely common. Increased sun exposure and/or the use of vitamin D supplements is required in order to achieve a blood vitamin D level of between 100 and 150 nmol/L 40 and 60 ng/mL).

Co Enzyme Q10: This is a fat soluble compound that your body manufactures, and you also consume in your diet. Co enzyme Q10 is required in high amounts by the mitochondria in your cells. The mitochondria need co enzyme Q10 in order to manufacture energy. The midpiece of sperm cells contains extremely high quantities of mitochondria, which are required to give the sperm energy to swim and help them swim in the correct manner. All men with compromised sperm motility require co enzyme Q10. Co enzyme Q10 is also a powerful antioxidant that protects the sperm cell membrane from oxidative damage (free radical damage).

Most cells of your body have the ability to manufacture co enzyme Q10, but this ability is impaired by poor health, stress and nutrient deficiencies; particularly vitamin B6 deficiency. Food provides very small amounts of this nutrient; meat, poultry and fish are the richest sources. Men with infertility require a co enzyme Q10 supplement of between 100 and 150 milligrams per day, taken with food.

Zinc: Healthy semen contains fairly high levels of zinc. Deficiency can lead to lower testosterone levels and this results in low sperm counts and a reduced ability of sperm to mature correctly. Zinc deficiency can promote the development of anti-sperm antibodies in men, and supplementation can correct this.[138] Zinc supplementation can increase sperm count, sperm motility and morphology and greatly increase the chance of conception.[139] Good food sources of zinc include oysters, beef, pork and chicken. Cashews, almonds, pumpkin seeds and peanuts contain small quantities. Men with infertility require a supplement containing 60 milligrams of elemental zinc per day. Zinc is best taken on an empty stomach.

Vitamin C: Deficiency of vitamin C increases free radical damage to sperm DNA. This is particularly a problem in older men (older than 40), men who smoke and men in occupations that expose them to toxic substances. Research has shown that vitamin C protects the DNA inside sperm from free radical damage, and improves the count, motility and morphology of sperm. Vitamin C also reduces the risk of birth defects. The membrane surrounding sperm cells is very rich in polyunsaturated fatty acids. These fats are very delicate and susceptible to harm caused by free radicals (oxidative damage).[140] An adequate intake of vitamin C helps to prevent this damage. Vitamin C is found in all fresh fruit and vegetables; however men wishing to conceive should take between 2 and 3 grams of vitamin C in supplement form each day.

B vitamins: All of the B group vitamins are essential for optimum fertility, however vitamin B9 (also known as folic acid) and vitamin B12 are the most important. Both of these vitamins are required for correct DNA replication. Mistakes in DNA replication cause abnormal cells and increase the risk of birth defects and cancer in the offspring. Vitamin B12 has improved sperm count in clinical trials. [141]. Research conducted on rats has shown that vitamin B12 deficiency produces lower sperm counts and increased sperm abnormalities.[142]

You are probably well aware that folic acid (vitamin B9) reduces the risk of neural tube defects in infants if a woman takes it before and during pregnancy. Well folic acid is vital for men as well because it is required for the production of normal healthy sperm. Research has shown that both fertile and infertile men experience an improvement in their sperm count when they take a folic acid supplement.[143] You can have a blood test to check your body's level of vitamins B12 and B9. You can also have a blood test for a substance called homocysteine. If it is raised, you are probably deficient in vitamin B12, B9 and B6. Vitamin B12 is found in animal foods, therefore vegetarians are commonly deficient. Folic acid is found in foliage; therefore green leafy vegetables are a great source of this nutrient. Men who are deficient in these vitamins should supplement with 1000 micrograms of vitamin B12 per day and 500 micrograms of folic acid.

Vitamin E: This vitamin is a fat soluble antioxidant and it reduces oxidative damage to sperm, and improves sperm motility.[144] Vitamin E helps to protect the delicate fatty acids in the sperm cell membrane, as well as the DNA inside sperm from damage. A study using a combination of antioxidants, including vitamin E showed that it improved ICSI outcomes.[145] Vitamin E is found in oily foods such as extra virgin olive oil, nuts, seeds and avocados. It is also available in supplement form. The best way to take vitamin E is as mixed tocopherols.

L-carnitine: This is a substance made in your body from the amino acid lysine. Poor health and nutrient deficiencies can impair the production of carnitine. Carnitine has a number of benefits in the body, including providing energy for testes and sperm cells. It is required in large quantities by the mitochondria in sperm cells, to help them swim vigorously. Several studies have shown that fertile men have far higher quantities of carnitine in their semen than infertile men.[146] L-carnitine or acetyl L-carnitine can be taken in supplement form at a dose of 500 milligrams to 2 grams per day.

Calcium: You probably don't associate calcium with healthy sperm but it is a key component of semen and provides nourishment for sperm. Research has shown that low calcium levels in semen are associated with fertility problems in men.[147] A calcium supplement is not always necessary for men with fertility problems because it should be easy enough to get adequate calcium from diet alone. Bones are an excellent source of calcium, therefore canned salmon or sardines provide lots of calcium. See page 161 for foods rich in calcium. It is best to avoid cow's milk.

Omega 3 fats: Research has shown that infertile men have lower levels of omega 3 fats in their sperm than fertile men. The ratio of omega 6 to omega 3 fats was also found to be higher in infertile men. Omega 6 fats increase inflammation and omega 3 fats dampen down inflammation. According to researchers from the Shahid Beheshti University in Tehran, Iran, "A high proportion of omega 6 fatty acids in the spermatozoa is a distinctive feature of infertile men. There is a growing body of evidence that the fatty acid composition of sperm membranes determines their physiological Characteristics". The Western world as a whole is suffering a severe deficiency of omega 3 fats, and poor sperm health is just one more manifestation of this. Men with infertility need to take a high strength fish oil supplement providing approximately 1200 mg of DHA and 1800 mg of EPA.

Daily ejaculation

Research has shown that if a man ejaculates daily, the quality of his sperm improves. His sperm count will be lower; however the sperm will be fresher and less likely to suffer with genetic damage. In a study of 118 Sydney men with higher than normal levels of sperm damage, 81 percent of the men experienced an average decrease in sperm DNA damage of 12 percent after ejaculating daily for seven days. This was in comparison to levels of DNA damage after three days of abstinence.[148] Quality is more important than quantity. A better quality sperm will produce a healthier child. The longer sperm is left to sit around in the testes, the more likely it is to undergo free radical damage.

Avoid long distance bicycle riding

A study from Spain has shown that triathletes who did the most cycling training had the worst sperm quality. The authors of the study suggested that this may be due to localized heat produced by wearing tight shorts, or irritation and compression to the testes from the bicycle saddle.[149] There are saddles commercially available that reduce pressure on the testes and penis.

Minimize exposure to environmental chemicals and radiation: This is covered in detail in chapter 9.

12. IVF: Maximizing outcomes

We are aware that many of you may have tried IVF or other assisted reproductive technologies in the past, or are contemplating using them in the future. We use the term assisted reproductive technology because it encompasses not only IVF, but also intrauterine insemination (IUI), ICSI (intracytoplasmic sperm injection) and other techniques. The vast majority of recommendations we have made in this book are compatible with these techniques, and indeed will improve your chances of success. The healthier you are as a couple, the better your chances of having a healthy child; whether that is naturally, or with the help of modern technology.

In this chapter we will explain the basics of the commonly used assisted reproductive technologies, so you have a better understanding of how they work and you can make a more informed decision. We strongly believe that IVF is overused, and in the vast majority of cases there are safe, inexpensive and effective alternatives available. All too often the real reasons behind a couple's infertility are never investigated fully; they are labeled as unexplained infertility; or worse, told the problem is genetic, and therefore nothing can be done, so IVF is the only option. Hopefully by reading this book you are now aware of the myriad factors that can impair fertility and that in most cases they can be rectified.

Worldwide increase in the use of assisted reproductive technologies (ARTs)

IVF has been in use for the last 30 years and approximately 3.5 million children have been conceived through this process. In Australia in that time there have been more than 85 thousand successful IVF births. According to Professor Michael Chapman, of IVF Australia, one in 29 Australian children is conceived using artificial reproduction technology. The average age of a woman using IVF is 36.5 years. According to the Australian Institute of Health and Welfare, use of IVF has grown by ten percent annually in recent years. The average success rate in 2007 was 17 percent per cycle. More than one percent of infants born in the USA are conceived through the use of assisted reproductive technology.

Ovulation induction

Ovulation induction medication is commonly referred to as fertility drugs. These drugs are used to stimulate the follicles in your ovaries, so that multiple eggs are produced in one menstrual cycle. The medications also control the time that you ovulate. This is very handy because sexual intercourse or intrauterine insemination or IVF procedures can be scheduled at the time you are most likely to conceive. There are some risks associated with the use of these drugs; the most common ones are multiple births and the development of ovarian cysts. A rare but serious side effect is ovarian hyperstimulation syndrome. Symptoms include difficulty breathing, severe pain in the pelvis, abdomen and chest, bloating and vomiting. Most IVF clinics now use lower doses of fertility drugs than in the past; therefore this potential side effect is becoming less common. The most commonly used ovulation induction drugs are clomiphene citrate, FSH injections, metformin and bromocriptine.

Clomiphene citrate (Clomid or Serophene)

These tablets are commonly used by women who have normal fallopian tubes, their partners have normal sperm, but the women rarely or never ovulate. They are a common first resort because they are inexpensive and are easy to use, compared to injections. Clomiphene is a synthetic hormone that behaves as an anti-estrogen. Therefore it tricks the pituitary gland in your brain to manufacture more FSH (follicle stimulating hormone). This stimulates the development of several ovarian follicles in one cycle. Your FSH level becomes much higher than you could ever naturally produce and this is intended to increase the number of eggs that mature and become available for fertilization. A course of clomiphene tablets is given for five days; typically from days 2 to 6 or 5 to 9 of your menstrual cycle.

Because these tablets block the effects of estrogen in your body, they can have side effects. The most common side effects include vaginal dryness, hot flushes and thickening of the cervical mucus. Some women notice mood changes, irritability, bloating, dizziness, a skin rash, blurry vision or breast tenderness. These symptoms are short lived and pass soon after you stop taking the tablets. Because clomiphene is an anti-estrogen drug, it thickens your cervical mucus and changes the lining of your uterus. Ironically, both of those factors reduce the chance of fertilization and conception. Therefore clomiphene has a pregnancy rate of five to ten percent per cycle, or 35 to 40 percent if used for a period of six months. Therefore, most women are advised to use clomiphene for a period of six months, unless they fall pregnant sooner. Some research has indicated that using clomiphene for 12 months or longer increases the risk of ovarian cancer.

Approximately ten percent of women using clomiphene will experience multiple pregnancy; most commonly twins. Triplets occur in roughly one in 400 births. You may consider a multiple birth a blessing; however it is important to remember that the risk of pregnancy complications is greater in women carrying twins or more embryos. Clomiphene also increases the risk of ovarian cysts. In most cases they resolve themselves, however in rare instances the cysts may cause internal bleeding, or they could twist and require immediate surgery.

Women who conceive through the use of clomiphene are at increased risk of suffering a miscarriage; particularly women with polycystic ovarian syndrome. There are two possible ways in which clomiphene may increase the risk of miscarriage: 1) It can force the development of an egg that contains chromosome abnormalities and would never have developed on its own because it can't sustain a pregnancy. 2) Because it acts as an anti-estrogen, it impairs the proper development of the uterine lining, making it more thin and inhospitable to a developing embryo. This is more likely to occur in slim women who naturally have lower estrogen levels anyway.

FSH and Human Chorionic Gonadotropin injections

Follicle stimulating hormone injections are given in order to promote multiple follicle development in the ovaries, so that several eggs are available for use in IVF. The FSH used is identical to what the body makes; it is just used in much higher doses. It is used as an injection that you self administer into your muscle each evening. The injection looks similar to what a diabetic uses to inject insulin. The two brands of FSH injections are Gonal-F and Puregon. You will be closely monitored with blood tests and ultrasounds to make sure ovarian follicles are developing properly and to measure their size.

When the follicles are the right size (as measured by ultrasound), you will be given an injection of human chorionic gonadotropin (hCG). Human chorionic gonadotropin is normally produced by the placenta during pregnancy, but it is structurally very similar to LH (luteinizing hormone), which every woman makes at the middle of her menstrual cycle. When hCG is injected into a non-pregnant woman, it acts in the same way as LH. It has the advantage of lasting longer in the body, and thus has a more reliable and consistent effect. The hCG injection triggers ovulation. The brand names of hCG injections are Pregnyl and Ovidrel.

This method of ovulation induction generally always causes the development of several mature eggs. Intercourse should be avoided because the risk of multiple pregnancy is extremely high. Therefore the ripe eggs are usually collected and saved for use in IVF. The risk of having twins with FSH injections is approximately 20 percent, and triplets or higher in five percent of cases. Side effects associated with FSH injections are minimal for most women and usually consist of bloating and mood changes. The pregnancy success rate is ten to 20 percent per cycle, increasing to 40 to 50 percent if used over six months. Success rates are lower in women aged over 38.

Metformin

Metformin is a medication commonly used in type 2 diabetes, but it can also be successfully used in women with polycystic ovarian syndrome, insulin resistance, or obese women to promote ovulation. The majority of women with these conditions have elevated blood levels of the hormone insulin, however their bodies do not respond to insulin properly. Elevated insulin inhibits ovarian follicles from developing properly and can prevent the release of an egg (ovulation). Metformin works by making the cells of your body more sensitive to insulin, therefore blood insulin levels eventually fall. This increases the chance of ovulation.

In the vast majority of cases, metformin is not wildly effective at all. Weight loss, exercise and a lower carbohydrate eating plan are much more successful over the long term for helping obese women and women with PCOS ovulate regularly. Metformin can cause nausea or diarrhea. It also promotes vitamin B12 deficiency. This is a problem for women wishing to conceive because vitamin B12 works with folate to reduce the risk of neural tube defects. It is also important for protecting the chromosomes inside your eggs from abnormalities, thus reducing the risk of passing on genetic problems to your children. Women who take metformin must have their blood levels of vitamin B12 monitored regularly. Brand names of metformin are Diabex and Diaformin.

Bromocriptine

This medication is commonly used in women with a pituitary tumor that secretes excess prolactin. Prolactin is the hormone that promotes breast cells to produce milk after birth. However, it is normal for your pituitary gland to manufacture small amounts of prolactin all the time. In some women, a pituitary tumor stimulates far too much prolactin to be produced, and this inhibits ovulation. The medication bromocriptine is usually very effective for keeping prolactin levels under control in these women, and therefore enables ovulation to occur. When you are pregnant, it is normal for your pituitary gland to increase in size by approximately 30 percent. This can be a problem in women who already have an enlarged pituitary gland due to a prolactin secreting tumor.

Intra-uterine insemination

This method is often used as a first resort procedure if a couple have not been able to achieve natural conception. It is used in couples where there are no known problems with sperm quality or fallopian tube problems. It can be used in cases where the man suffers with a low sperm count, or the sperm have poor motility. This procedure can increase the chance of successful conception because the sperm do not have far to travel; they are deposited right near the egg in the uterus. Intra-uterine insemination is often used in cases of unexplained infertility as an initial option, before IVF is attempted. It can be used in women who do not ovulate each month, because the ovulation inducing drug clomiphene is usually given to a woman in this procedure.

Explanation of the process

You will usually be asked to take the drug clomiphene from day 3 to day 7 of your menstrual cycle. On day 8 or 9 of your cycle you will be given an ultrasound of your pelvis to make sure that your ovaries contain developing follicles. At that stage you will be asked to use FSH (follicle stimulating hormone) injections daily to promote development of those follicles. The aim is for you to produce one or two mature eggs at the time of ovulation, so that one of them can be fertilized by a sperm when they are injected into your cervix. The developing follicles in your ovaries are regularly monitored via ultrasound scans, which you will have every second or third day. Urine ovulation test kits are also often used to monitor your hormone levels and make sure everything is progressing according to plan.

Once it has been confirmed that you have ovulated, your partner's sperm is injected into your uterus through a narrow plastic tube that is inserted into your uterus. Either your partner's sperm or donor sperm can be used. The sperm are "washed" before they are injected. This means they are separated from the seminal fluid, analyzed under a microscope and filtered so that only normal looking sperm are introduced into your body.

This technique is not hugely successful; it has a success rate of between ten and twenty percent per cycle. Some researchers argue that it is no more successful than regular sexual intercourse. The women most likely to benefit from this procedure are those with polycystic ovarian syndrome, obesity, insulin resistance or other conditions that prevent regular ovulation, due to the use of clomiphene which induces ovulation.

IVF (In Vitro Fertilization)

In vitro fertilization is basically the process whereby the sperm and egg are joined together in a laboratory (in vitro), instead of inside your fallopian tubes. The development, maturation and release of eggs is completely controlled with the use of hormones. Ironically, the process often begins with placing a woman on the contraceptive pill in order to inhibit natural ovulation and enable it to be timed and controlled more easily. The next step is usually to self administer FSH injections, in order to promote development of several ovarian follicles. Ultrasounds and blood tests are regularly performed, in order to monitor the number of ovarian follicles, their size and location. Sometimes you may be given additional drugs to prevent premature ovulation. They can be administered as a nasal spray or injection.

When the follicles are considered ripe, you are given a hCG injection to trigger ovulation, and then approximately 37 hours later your eggs are retrieved. You will be given a general anaesthetic and your eggs may be collected transvaginally or laparoscopically. After your eggs are collected, your partner's sperm are added to them approximately four hours later, as this most closely mimics what happens in nature. A semen sample is obtained from your partner on the day your eggs are to be retrieved.

Sperm are added to each egg and allowed to incubate overnight under controlled laboratory conditions. The next day each egg is checked for fertilization. If fertilization has not occurred, the eggs are re-inseminated, or intracytoplasmic sperm injection (ICSI) is offered. This procedure is explained in the following section. If fertilization has been successful, between three and five days after the eggs were inseminated, the divided embryo is transferred into your uterus using a fine catheter that is inserted through your cervix. If the embryo survives to day five (the blastocyst stage), there is a good chance it will go on to develop into a healthy baby.

The critical factors required for an embryo to make it to day five are adequate energy and normal chromosomes. The embryo obtains energy from the mitochondria inside your egg, until the placenta forms. Therefore you need healthy mitochondria for successful IVF.

In most instances, only one embryo is transferred, in order to minimize the chance of multiple pregnancy. In women who are older than 38 years, some IVF clinics will transfer two embryos, in order to maximise the chance of conception. The risk of complications is increased when more than one embryo is transferred. You may have additional embryos frozen for later use. It is possible to have an IVF cycle without the use of any hormones. This is called a natural cycle, and just one egg is collected for use in the laboratory. The main purpose of using hormones is to ensure ovulation occurs and to gather several eggs, thus increasing the chances of successful conception.

A blood test is done to confirm pregnancy seven to ten days after the embryo has been transferred into your uterus, to make sure it has implanted properly and the pregnancy is progressing. It is very common to have a little bleeding or spotting after the embryo transfer and this is not a bad sign.

Intracytoplasmic Sperm Injection (ICSI)

In this procedure a single sperm is injected into a single egg. It is used when conventional IVF has failed, or when there are sperm problems such as poor sperm motility and morphology or when sperm antibodies are present. A sperm is chosen based on its normal shape and size. Generally the DNA inside the sperm is not analyzed unless you ask for it to be done.

Due to the growing problem of male infertility, ICSI has now overtaken conventional IVF as the most common assisted reproductive procedure performed in Europe and most other parts of the world. ICSI is a relatively new procedure; the first baby born this way was in 1992. Traditional IVF requires more than half a million sperm for a good chance of fertilization, while ICSI requires only one sperm.

Other forms of assisted reproduction

Gamete intrafallopian transfer (GIFT).

In this procedure eggs are removed from a woman's ovary, combined with sperm and both are injected into a fallopian tube. Hopefully fertilization then takes place inside the fallopian tube. For some people GIFT is more morally acceptable than IVF.

Zygote intrafallopian transfer (ZIFT)

In this procedure IVF is used to achieve fertilization but the fertilized egg is transferred into a fallopian tube the day after IVF. This means the fertilized egg is transferred at the earliest stage of conception, before the cells have divided (zygote stage).

Risks associated with assisted reproductive technology

There are real and significant risks associated with these

procedures. Dr Alastair Sutcliffe of the Institute of Child Health at University College London and Professor Michael Ludwig of the Centre for Reproductive Medicine and Gynecologic Endocrinology in Hamburg performed a review of 3,980 articles in scientific and medical journals published between 1980 and 2005. They found some startling results.

The research showed there are significantly greater risks of long term health problems for children conceived through artificial means such as IVF and ICSI. The researchers have advised that these children should be monitored well into adulthood, as there is no long term data available tracking their health.

Their analysis of the research showed that there is:

- 55 percent greater risk of pre-eclampsia
- 20 to 34 percent greater risk of miscarriage
- 155 percent greater risk of stillbirth
- 170 to 200 percent increased risk of very low birth weight[150]

Other research conducted on 17 thousand Australian women has found children born through IVF are delivered via caesarean section 44 percent of the time, compared to 28 percent in children conceived naturally.[151] Other studies have shown that children conceived through IVF visit hospitals significantly more often than children conceived naturally.

Increased risk of birth defects

Children born through IVF are at significantly increased risk of birth defects, according to the largest study of its kind. They are particularly prone to being born with heart defects and abnormalities in the reproductive organs. IVF children are also at higher risk of cerebral palsy and autism and infertility. The risk of infertility is particularly high for boys born to infertile fathers. Scientists carried out a survey of 33 French infertility clinics and collected data on more than 15 thousand births between the years 2003 and 2007. They discovered that 4.24 percent of children born through IVF had some kind of congenital deformity, compared to a rate of between two and three percent for children conceived naturally.

According to Dr Viot, a clinical geneticist at the Maternite Port Royal Hospital in Paris, "a malformation rate of this magnitude is a public health issue". She said there are a range of possible explanations, including infertility itself, ovarian stimulation, the maturing of eggs in a laboratory, or the intracytoplasmic sperm injection process.[152]

Along with an increased risk of genetic problems being handed down from parents to children through IVF, there is also an increased risk of passing on what are known as imprinting disorders. There are several conditions that come under this category, including Beckwith-Wiedemann syndrome and Angelman syndrome, Silver-Russell syndrome, maternal hypomethylation syndrome, and retinoblastoma. Some research has linked the use of assisted reproductive technology with a higher incidence of these disorders in offspring.[153]

Researchers believe that epigenetic disorders can be passed on to children who are conceived through the use of IVF. This means that the laboratory process involved in IVF can change the way genes inside your eggs behave, in a way to potentially cause health problems in children. These changes occur due to insufficient DNA methylation in eggs. The behavior of the genes inside eggs is thought to be more susceptible to epigenetic disorders than the DNA inside sperm because sperm are fully mature by the time they are used in IVF, whereas eggs are still ripening during the IVF process.

DNA methylation is a process that occurs inside all of your cells all the time; in fact it occurs billions of times every second. Methylation is a process that repairs the DNA inside your cells continually. You need optimal levels of B vitamins in your body to keep methylation running smoothly. Inadequate B vitamins before and during any pregnancy increases the risk of genetic disorders such as Down syndrome, spina bifida and miscarriage. These risks are heightened in IVF pregnancies. IVF pregnancies are also at increased risk of epigenetic changes, where the genes remain the same, but they behave in a problematic way to potentially cause disease in children born this way.

We believe these disturbing figures are most likely a result of poor quality egg and sperm, joined together by force to create a child with compromised health. Mother Nature is wise, and if you or your partner are suffering with compromised fertility, there is a reason for this. Ideally both of you would improve your diet and lifestyle and address all underlying health issues before attempting conception. That way you will be passing on only the best quality egg and sperm possible, both of which form the basis of your child's lifelong health. Intracytoplasmic sperm injection seems to be more related to health problems in children than standard IVF, probably because the sperm clearly suffer with abnormalities if they are not able to penetrate the egg on their own.

Optimizing health outcomes in children born through IVF and other assisted reproductive technologies

A study conducted by Foresight, which is the Association for Pre-conceptual Health care in the UK found that couples going through IVF are up to 47 percent more successful if they use a pre-conceptual health care program first. It is fantastic to know that you have the power to influence IVF outcomes so profoundly. With the right diet and nutrients, not only will your IVF cycle be more likely to be successful; you can also reduce the risk of negative health outcomes in your children.

If you do decide to undergo IVF, it is vital that you play an active role in your health because IVF does absolutely nothing to improve the health of the egg or sperm. It also does nothing to improve the health of your pregnancy or your child. Therefore, please follow the diet guidelines on chapter 8 of this book. They are equally applicable whether you are conceiving naturally or through assisted reproductive technology. In addition, here are some strategies for increasing your chances of success through IVF.

Strategies for increasing your chances of a healthy pregnancy through IVF

Improve sperm health

Poor sperm health is a common cause of IVF failure; this is evident with the increased reliance on intra-cytoplasmic sperm injection (ICSI). Even sperm that look normal under a microscope and swim normally can contain high levels of DNA fragmentation (DNA damage). That is why it is essential for your partner to have a sperm chromatin structure assay test of his sperm to check for levels of DNA damage if you are having difficulties conceiving. This is especially important if your partner is 40 years of age or older, and if he is in an occupation notorious for chemical exposure. See chapter 11 for more information about optimizing sperm health.

Improve the health of your mitochondria

Mitochondria are the energy generating structures inside all of your cells. The mitochondria inside your eggs are what provides energy to your developing embryo once the egg and sperm have been joined and before the placenta starts to form. Once the sperm has penetrated the egg its midpiece and tail fall away, so that only the head of the sperm fuses with the egg.

Therefore all the mitochondria responsible for providing the rapidly dividing cells with energy come from the woman. Mitochondria are highly sensitive to free radical damage; therefore you need a lot of antioxidants inside your body to protect them. Mitochondria contain numerous inner cell membranes which are composed of delicate fatty acids. These fatty acids are highly susceptible to oxidation. Along with antioxidants, mitochondria have a high requirement for omega 3 fats and magnesium.

Maximise methylation

As mentioned previously, methylation is the process your body uses to repair DNA. This process is heavily reliant on B vitamins and is influenced by several lifestyle factors. A blood test for homocysteine will give you some indication of how well methylation functions in your body; high levels of homocysteine are a definite indicator of a problem and you should not attempt to conceive until this is resolved. A blood test called a full blood count can reveal deficiency of B vitamins; having abnormally large red blood cells (macrocytic anemia) can indicate poor methylation. Vitamins B6, B12 and folate are the most important nutrients for methylation and it is important to take them in supplement form to guarantee you receive enough.

Excess sugar, coffee, cigarettes and alcohol can all deplete you of B vitamins, but they are not substances you'll be consuming while trying to fall pregnant anyway. People with poor digestion and particularly insufficient hydrochloric acid in the stomach do not absorb vitamin B12 as well, and this needs to be addressed. Increase your intake of dark green leafy vegetables. They are an excellent source of folate. Examples include bok choy and all Asian leafy greens, kale, spinach, silverbeet, watercress, dandelion leaves, rocket and parsley.

Increase your intake of foods rich in vitamin B6, such as sunflower seeds, bananas, hazelnuts, salmon and chicken.

Increase your intake of foods high in vitamin B12, such as fish, beef, chicken and eggs. Vegetarians and vegans must take a B12 supplement.

Minimize your exposure to chemicals

This is essential for all couples attempting conception, however studies have shown that exposure to environmental chemicals reduces the chances of IVF success. See chapter 9 for comprehensive information on this topic.

Address immune system problems

Research has shown that women with auto-antibodies in their bloodstream have poor IVF outcomes. If you have an autoimmune disease, allergies or excess inflammation in your body, you are at risk of having your immune cells destroy the embryo once it is transferred into your uterus. Follow our recommendations for reducing inflammation on chapter 5.

Use natural progesterone

Progesterone will help to hold the pregnancy until the placenta is well formed and can produce sufficient progesterone on its own. Progesterone will also help to dampen down an overactive immune system and reduce the risk of your immune cells destroying the embryo. Progesterone supplementation in the form of pessaries, troches or cream should be used for the first 16 weeks of pregnancy. Progesterone is commonly used in IVF but it is usually not used for long enough. See page 49 for more information on the importance of progesterone.

Recommended supplements for women undergoing IVF

The following supplements will help to increase your chances of success:

- B vitamins. Folic acid should be taken at a dose of 500 to

1000 micrograms daily. Higher amounts are required for some women. Some women need to take an activated form of folic acid called folinic acid. This bypasses some of the steps in folic acid activation. Vitamin B6 should be taken in a dose of 250 mg per day. Vitamin B12 should be taken at a dose of 500 to 1000 mcg per day. Some people don't absorb oral vitamin B12 well, therefore a sublingual spray or B12 injections may be required.

- Magnesium in a dose of 400 mg daily. It is easier to obtain high strength magnesium in powder form.
- Vitamin D in a dose of between 1000 and 5000 IU per day. The dose you require will depend on the time of year and several other factors. Blood tests will confirm what dose you require.
- Fish oil will improve the health of your mitochondria and reduce inflammation in your body. The dose should provide roughly 1200 mg of DHA and 1800 mg of EPA.
- Selenium will help to reduce chromosomal abnormalities in the egg and sperm. The dose is 200 mcg daily.

You may require other supplements, depending on your current state of health. It is best to consult a naturopath for personalized help.

Supplements to avoid during IVF

It is important to avoid taking all herbs during this time, as many herbs have hormone modulating effects. Even herbs that are not traditionally used for their hormonal properties can have a subtle effect on your hormone levels.

It is also important to avoid all blood thinning supplements approximately one week before your eggs are collected. You can resume those supplements a week after the embryo has been transferred to your uterus. Blood thinning supplements include fish oil, flaxseed oil, co enzyme Q10 and vitamin E.

Regarding medication and IVF, as a general rule if the substance is safe to take during pregnancy, it is safe to use during IVF. Acetaminophen and codeine are safe to take, but avoid aspirin and ibuprofen. Some women need to take a low dose of aspirin to reduce the risk of blood clots and this is acceptable under medical supervision.

Conclusion

We sincerely hope that reading this book will enable you to uncover the factors that are impairing your fertility and give you the tools to resolve them. Knowledge is power, and the more you understand about your body and what is required for healthy fertility, the better able you will be to resolve it. The healthier you and your partner are before conceiving a child, the healthier your child is likely to be.

Please try not to rush; use this book and take the time to get healthy and fertile. It will not provide the best outcomes for you or your offspring to rush into assisted reproductive techniques whilst you are highly stressed and/or suffering with undetected and/or untreated health problems. Thankfully these conditions are often easy to overcome; but you need to recognize them before they interfere with your pregnancy outcome.

The healthier you are now, the easier your pregnancy and labor is likely to be. By improving the health of the parents, it is our aim to create a healthier future generation.

If you have questions after reading this book, we would love you to get in contact with us. We offer a number of personalized services that you and your partner may wish to utilize. For more information phone Dr Cabot's Health Advisory Line in Australia on 02 4655 8855 or the United States of America on 623 334 3232 or email contact@weightcontroldoctor.com

We also have clinics where you can see a naturopath for a personalized consultation. Phone us or see our website www. weightcontroldoctor.com.au for contact details.

Glossary

Acrosome
A cap-like structure that sits on the head of the sperm. It contains enzymes that help the sperm to digest the wall of the egg, in order to allow the sperm to fertilize the egg.

Adenomyosis
A condition where endometrial tissue (lining of the uterus) grows into the muscle wall of the uterus (myometrium). An isolated area of adenomyosis can be hard to distinguish from a fibroid on an ultrasound. Sometimes adenomyosis is widespread through the uterus. Typically the condition causes period pain, but blood cannot drain out through the vagina, therefore periods are usually not

heavy.

Adhesions
Scar tissue, usually caused by endometriosis, infection or previous surgery. The scar tissue can interfere with the function of the ovaries, fallopian tubes or uterus. Microsurgery can be used to remove adhesions if they are interfering with fertility.

Amenorrhea
Absence of menstrual periods.

Androgens
Male sex hormones; primarily testosterone and androstenedione.

Anolulation
Absence of ovulation.

Anticardiolipin antibody
Antibodies directed against a component of cell membranes and mitochondrial membranes. Women who produce these antibodies have blood that clots too quickly, and this can cause miscarriage.

Antinuclear antibody (ANA)
This antibody causes inflammation in the body and potentially in the uterus, where it can cause infertility or miscarriage. It is usually present in women with lupus, but can be present in any autoimmune disease.

Antiphospholipid antibody
These antibodies are made by the immune system and attack phospholipids, which are molecules on the surface of cells. Women with antiphospholipid antibodies have a high tendency to form blood clots. During pregnancy, blood clots around the uterus can cut off blood supply to the developing baby and lead to miscarriage. The antibodies can also cause the placenta to attach too weakly to the uterus. The conventional treatment is to give these women baby aspirin and heparin (a blood thinner) before conception and through pregnancy.

Autoimmune
Autoimmune disease is where the body produces antibodies or immune cells that attack and destroy the body's own organs and tissues. Examples of autoimmune diseases are systemic lupus erythematosus, rheumatoid arthritis and Hashimoto's thyroiditis.

Azoospermia
An absence of sperm in semen.

Blastocyst
An early stage of development of the embryo, usually five days after fertilization. A blastocyst consists of between 75 and 100 cells. This is usually the stage that an embryo is transferred to the uterus in IVF.

Chlamydia
A sexually transmitted infection that is capable of causing infertility in women, typically by causing scarring and blockage of the fallopian tubes. In men untreated infection can cause blockage of the tubes that carry sperm from the testes to the outside. Chlamydia is treated by giving antibiotics to both partners.

Chorionic villous sampling
A procedure done at approximately nine weeks of pregnancy where a catheter is inserted through the vagina and a small sample of cells is taken from the placenta. It is done to check for genetic and biochemical abnormalities. This test is done earlier in pregnancy than amniocentesis.

Chromosomes
These are rod-shaped structures (genes), made up of DNA and located in the nucleus of cells. Your cells contain 23 pairs of chromosomes; one of the pair came from your mother, and the other came from your father. The sex chromosomes are called X and Y chromosomes. Girls have two X chromosomes and boys have one X and one Y chromosome.

Clomiphene (brand names Clomid and Serophene)
A drug commonly used in infertility clinics to induce the ovaries to produce more mature eggs. It blocks the action of estrogen, therefore your brain believes there is not enough estrogen in your body. Consequently your brain produces higher amounts of FSH (follicle stimulating hormone) and this stimulates the maturation of several eggs.

Congenital
Meaning present from birth. Usually refers to an abnormality. It can be caused by a genetic problem or environmental trigger.

Corpus luteum
The remaining egg sac in the ovary after the egg has been released at ovulation. The corpus luteum produces progesterone in the second half of the menstrual cycle.

Cryptorchidism
Undescended testes. Approximately three percent of full term and 30 percent of premature infant boys are born with one or both undescended testes. Men who are born with this condition have a higher rate of infertility and testicular cancer.

Cytokine
A chemical made by immune cells, fat cells and possibly other tissues that communicates with other cells of your immune system. Cytokines are involved in fighting infections, or rejection of something by your body (such as an embryo or organ transplant). Cytokines promote inflammation and free radical damage in the body.

Dysmenorrhoea
Painful menstruation.

Ectopic pregnancy
Occurs when the embryo implants in the wrong location (not the uterus). May occur in a fallopian tube, cervix, ovary or peritoneal cavity.

Embryo
The earliest stage of development of a baby, beginning at fertilization.

Endocrine disruptor
An environmental substance that interferes with normal hormone action in the body. Implicated in the development of endometriosis, uterine fibroids and low sperm counts.

Endometriosis
A disease where the lining of the uterus (endometrium) grows and menstruates in abnormal locations in the body, such as the ovaries, fallopian tubes, bowel, bladder or abdominal cavity. Endometriosis can cause infertility.

Endometrium
The lining of the uterus, which is shed each month as menstrual bleeding. In the second half of the menstrual cycle the endometrium thickens, so that it is a hospitable location for implantation of the embryo if fertilization occurs.

Epididymis
Finely coiled tubes that lie next to the testes in the scrotum. These tubes connect the testes to the vas deferens. Sperm cells develop as they pass through these tubes.

Fibroid
A benign tumor in the muscular wall of the uterus. Fibroids can be located on the outside of the uterus, within the wall or grow into the cavity. They are more common with increasing age. Fibroids can lead to infertility or miscarriage.

Fetus
An unborn baby. From the time the embryo is fully formed until delivery.

Follicle Stimulating Hormone (FSH)
A hormone made by the pituitary gland of the brain which stimulates the ovaries to produce eggs and manufacture estrogen. In men FSH stimulates the testes to manufacture sperm.

Follicular phase
The first half of the menstrual cycle, from the first day of bleeding to ovulation.

Gonad
Refers to the ovaries or testes.

Heparin
A blood thinning drug that is given as an injection. It can prevent miscarriage in women who have a propensity to form blood clots.

Human chorionic gonadotropin (hCG)
Detection of this hormone is the basis of a blood test for pregnancy. hCG is produced by cells of the placenta and levels are high in early pregnancy. hCG is also given as an injection to women undergoing assisted reproductive technology, such as IVF in order to trigger ovulation. Typically women will ovulate 36 to 40 hours after this injection.

Hydrosalpinx
Blockage of a fallopian tube that causes it to swell and fill with fluid. Can result in infertility.

Hypothalamus
Part of the brain above and connected to the pituitary gland. It releases hormones that control the pituitary gland, which then controls the ovaries and testes.

Hysterosalpingogram (HSG)
An X ray that involves injection of a dye into the uterus and fallopian tubes. It enables a doctor to see the size and shape of your uterus and detect any abnormalities. The test can determine if the fallopian tubes are blocked.

Hysterosalpingo contrast sonography (HyCoSy)
A very similar but preferable test to a HSG because it uses ultrasound rather than X rays.

In vitro fertilization (IVF)
The fertilization of an egg by a sperm in a laboratory.

Intracytoplasmic sperm injection (ICSI)
A procedure sometimes carried out with IVF where a single sperm is injected into an egg by a doctor in the laboratory.

Intrauterine insemination (IUI)
A form of assisted reproduction where sperm are directly injected into the uterus with a catheter. The procedure can either be carried out with a woman's natural menstrual cycle, or with ovarian stimulation (using clomiphene tablets or FSH injections).

Karyotype
A test that determines the status of chromosomes after cells are grown in a tissue culture. The test is done in women and men when recurrent miscarriage is occurring. A normal female karyotype is 46 XX and for males it is 46 XY

Killer cells
A type of white blood cell that has the ability to destroy other cells. Sometimes natural killer cells destroy the placenta or embryo.

Laparoscopy
A minimally invasive surgical procedure where a long thin telescope-like instrument is inserted into the abdomen through an incision, usually in the navel. Sometimes additional incisions are also made, to allow other instruments to be inserted. A laparoscopy allows a doctor to diagnose abnormalities in the uterus, ovaries or fallopian tubes, particularly endometriosis. The procedure is also used to perform minor surgeries, such as removing endometriosis, ovarian cysts, scar tissue and ectopic pregnancies.

Leydig cells
Cells of the testes responsible for producing testosterone under the influence of luteinizing hormone.

Luteal phase
The second half of the menstrual cycle, beginning at ovulation and ending when menstrual bleeding starts.

Luteal phase defect
Insufficient progesterone production in the second half of the menstrual cycle. Can be caused by a variety of factors and typically results in infertility or miscarriage. Progesterone supplementation is effective for correcting luteal phase defects.

Luteinizing hormone (LH)
A hormone made by the pituitary gland of the brain that finishes the development of an egg and triggers ovulation. LH stimulates the corpus luteum to produce progesterone. In men LH stimulates the testes to produce testosterone.

Menorrhagia
Heavy menstrual bleeding.

Metformin
A medication commonly used for type 2 diabetes but also used in women with polycystic ovarian syndrome and insulin resistance. It helps to reduce androgens (male hormones), luteinizing hormone, insulin and helps with weight loss. It can help women who don't ovulate to ovulate more regularly.

Metrorrhagia
Bleeding between menstrual periods.

Mitochondria
Tiny structures inside cells that are responsible for generating energy.

Myomectomy
An operation to remove a myoma (uterine fibroid).

Myometrium
The muscular wall of the uterus.

Oestradiol (E2)
The most potent form of estrogen in the body. Women make three types of estrogen: Oestrone (E1), oestradiol (E2) and oestriol (E3).

Oligomenorrhoea
Infrequent menstrual periods.

Oocytes
Eggs produced by the ovaries.

Ovulation induction
The use of drugs to stimulate the development of follicles in the ovaries and stimulate ovulation. The most commonly used drugs are clomiphene, FSH and hCG. This procedure is used in women who do not ovulate, and also used in assisted reproductive technologies such as IVF.

Pituitary gland
A gland located at the base of the brain that is responsible for producing hormones that control the ovaries, testes, thyroid gland, adrenal glands and other organs. The pituitary gland makes the hormones FSH, LH, TSH and others.

Polycystic ovarian syndrome
A syndrome whereby many small cysts are present in the ovaries, along with symptoms of excess male hormones (androgens) such as acne, scalp hair loss, abdominal weight gain, excess facial and body hair and infrequent or absent menstruation. A common cause of infertility.

Pre-eclampsia
A condition occurring in late pregnancy marked by high blood pressure, fluid accumulation and the presence of albumin (protein) in the urine. There is reduced blood flow to the fetus, thereby placing it at risk of death. The condition usually results in pre-term delivery of the fetus. If left untreated, may progress to eclampsia (convulsions).

Premature ovarian failure
Also called early menopause. Cessation of menstruation before the age of 40. It is typically caused by autoimmune disease of the ovaries.

Progesterone
A hormone made by the ovaries in the second half of the menstrual cycle (after ovulation). Large quantities of progesterone are produced during pregnancy, first by the corpus luteum, and later by the placenta.

Prolactin
A hormone produced by the pituitary gland of the brain that stimulates breasts to produce milk. Tiny amounts of this hormone are made by women and men all the time, but very large quantities are produced after a woman gives birth. Sometimes a tumor on the pituitary gland can produce excessively high levels of prolactin and this can interfere with fertility.

Retrograde ejaculation
A disorder of ejaculation where instead of spurting out of the penis, semen spills upwards and into the bladder. Diabetes is the most common condition to produce this disorder.

Rh factor
Refers to a person's blood type. Approximately 15 percent of women lack the

Rh factor on their red blood cells, therefore they are called Rh negative. Women who do have the factor on their red blood cells are called Rh positive. Rh refers to Rhesus, since it was first discovered in Rhesus monkeys. If an Rh negative woman is pregnant with an Rh positive baby, she can make antibodies against the baby's red blood cells, thereby causing fetal death. This problem can be prevented by giving a pregnant woman Rh immunoglobulin.

Salpingitis
Inflammation of the fallopian tubes, most commonly caused by infection. Can lead to blockage of the tubes and infertility.

Sertoli cells
Cells in the testes that nourish the developing sperm cells.

Spermatozoon
A sperm cell. The plural is spermatozoa.

Sperm chromatin structure assay
A test done to check what percentage of sperm have damage to their DNA. A level lower than 15 percent is considered normal and should not impair fertility. This test is an optional add on to a semen analysis.

Spermatogenesis
Sperm cell production.

Testosterone
The main male sex hormone. Is typically elevated in women with polycystic ovarian syndrome.

Thrombophilia
An increased tendency to form blood clots. Can be caused by immune system disorders or inherited disorders. May increase the risk of infertility, miscarriage and stillbirth.

Thyroid stimulating hormone (TSH)
A hormone made by the pituitary gland of the brain that triggers the thyroid gland to manufacture hormones.

Transvaginal ultrasound
An ultrasound where a probe is inserted into the vagina. Used to check the health of the pelvic organs and to monitor the development of ovarian follicles with ovulation induction techniques or assisted reproductive technology, such as IVF.

Varicocele
A varicose vein in the scrotum. In some cases this can increase the temperature within the testes, thereby reducing sperm production and damaging already formed sperm. Can be surgically corrected.

Vas deferens
A long tube in men that transports sperm cells from the epididymis to the seminal vesicles. This tube may become blocked due to infection, thereby causing infertility. These tubes are cut when men have a vasectomy (there is a tube running from each testicle).

Vasovasostomy
Vasectomy reversal.

References

1. The fertility Society of Australia
2. Matarese G et al. Trends Mol Med 2003;9(5):223-228
3. The impact of endometriosis on infertility orgyn.com Issue 02-15 Feb 2010
4. Rier, S et al. Endometriosis in rhesus monkeys following chronic exposure to 2,3,7,8-Tetrachlorodibenzo-p-dioxin. Fundamental and Applied Toxicology 1993. 21:433-441
5. Rier S et al. Serum levels of TCDD and dioxin-like chemicals in rhesus monkeys chronically exposed to dioxin: correlation of increased serum PCB levels with endometriosis. Toxicological Sciences 2001. 59:147-159
6. Quaranta MG et al. Life Sci 2006;79(5):491-498
7. Mehmet Guney, et al. Regression of endometrial implants in a rat model of endometriosis treated with melatonin. Fertility & Sterility April 2008 Volume 89, issue 4
8. Missmer SA et al. A prospective study of dietary fat consumption and endometriosis risk. Hum Reprod. 2010 Mar 23
9. Chapkin RS, et al. Dietary docosahexaenoic and eicosapentaenoic acid: emerging mediators of inflammation. Prostaglandins Leukot Essent Fatty Acids 2009 Aug-Sep;81(2-3):187-91
10. Klatsky PC et al. Am J Obstet Gynecol 2008;198(4):357-366
11. M. Nathaniel Mead. From one womb to another: Early estrogenic exposures and later fibroid risk. Environ Health Perspect 118:a131
12. Green tea shows promise for uterine fibroids Natural Products Insider 25/01/2010
13. Polycystic Ovarian Syndrome Association of Australia
14. Eggers S et al. Anthropol Anz 2007;65(2):169-179
15. Dumesic et al 2007 Polycystic Ovary Syndrome and Oocyte Developmental Competence OG Survey 63:39.
16. Janssen OE. High prevalence of autoimmune thyroiditis in patients with polycystic ovary syndrome. Eur J Endocrin 150(3): 363-369
17. Forges, T., Monnier-Barbarino, P., Faure, G. C., and Bene, M.C.. Autoimmunity and antigenic targets in ovarian pathology. Human Reproduction Update, Vol.10, No.2 pp. 163±175, 2004
18. Yan HN, Wang CY, Sze CW et al. J Clin Psychopharmacol 2008; 28(3): 264-270
19. Wassermann EE, Nelson K et al. Am J Epidemiol 2008; 167(6):701-710
20. Negro R, Formoso G et al. Endocrinol Invest 2007; 30(1):3-8
21. Wartofsky L, Dickey RA. The evidence for a narrower thyrotropin reference range is compelling. J Clin Endocrinol Metab. 2005 Sep;90(9):5483-8
22. Weetman AP. Hypothyroidism: screening and subclinical disease. BMJ 1997;314:1175-8
23. Pasco JA, Henry MJ, Nicholson GC, et al. Vitamin D status of women in the Geelong Osteoporosis Study: association with diet and casual exposure to sunlight. Med J Aust 2001; 175: 401-405.

24. Sydney IVF

25. Stefano Guandalini MD Celiac disease does not cause infertility in the US. Or does it? The University of Chicago Celiac Disease Center. Winter 2008, vol 8, issue 1

26. Sher KS, Mayberry JF: Female fertility, obstetric and gynecological history in coeloac disease. A case control study. Digestion 1994;55(4):243-6

27. Martinelli P, Troncone R, et al. Celiac disease and unfovourable outcome of pregnancy. Gut 2000;46(3):332-5

28. Ciacci C et al. Celiac disease and pregnancy outcome. Am J Gastroenterol 1996;91(4):718-22

29. American Thyroid Association 80th Annual Meeting September 25, 2009.

30. The Australian Institute of Health and Welfare

31. Sausenthaler S, et al. Maternal diet during pregnancy in relation to eczema and allergic sensitization in the offspring at 2y of age. Am J Clin Nutr 2007;85:530-537

32. Furuhjelm C, et al. Fish oil supplementation in pregnancy and lactation may decrease the risk of infant allergy. Acta Paediatr 2009 Sep;98(9):1461-1467

33. Nwaru BI, et al. Maternal diet during pregnancy and allergic sensitization in the offspring by 5yrs of age: a prospective cohort study. Pediatr Allergy Immunol 2010 Feb;21(1Pt1):29-37

34. VassalloMF, et al. Potential mechanisms for the hypothesized link between sunshine, vitamin D and food allergy in children. J Allergy Clin Immunol 2010 Aug;126(2):217-222

35. Osborn DA, et al. Probiotics in infants for prevention of allergic disease and food hypersensitivity. Cochrane Database of Systematic Reviews 2007, Issue 4.

36. Sang-Cheol Bae, et al. Impaired antioxidant status and decreased dietary intake of antioxidants in patients with systemic lupus erythematosus Rheumatology International Volume 22, number 6, 238-243

37. The Journal of Clinical Endocrinology & Metabolism, Vol. 87, No. 4 1490-1498

38. www.health.gov.au

39. Hafner LM, McNeilly C. Future Microbiol 2008;3(1):67-77

40. Paavonen J. Eggert-Kruse W. Hum Reprod Update 1999;5(5):433-447

41. Abdulmedzhidova AG, Kurilo LF et al. Urologiia 2007; May-Jun (3):56-59

42. Gdoura R, Kchaou W et al. BMC Infectious Diseases 2007;7:129

43. Haggerty CL Curr Opin Infect Dis 2008;21(1):65-69

44. L.M. Bodnar, M.A. Krohn, H.N. Simhan "Maternal Vitamin D Deficiency Is Associated with Bacterial Vaginosis in the First Trimester of Pregnancy" Journal of Nutrition 8 April 2009, doi:10.3945/jn.108.103168

45. American Academy of Periodontology

46. American Academy of Periodontology

47. Baghurst KI, Droesti IE, Syrette JA, Record SJ, Baghurst PA, Buckley RA. Zinc and magnesium status of Australian adults. Nutr Res 1991; 11 : 23-32.

48. Prasad AS. Clinical, biochemical and nutritional spectrum of zinc defi ciency in human subjects, an update. Nutr Rev1983; 41(7) : 197.

49. Linus Pauling Institute Oregon State University

50. American Society for Reproductive Medicine

51. Miscarriage Support Auckland Inc

52. Piccinni MP, Beloni L, Livi C et al. Defective production of both leukemia inhibitory factor and type 2 T helper cytokines by decidual T cells in unexplained recurrent abortions. Nat Med 1998;4(9):1020-1024

53. Female veterinarians at risk of miscarriage from anaesthetic gases and pesticides, study suggests. Science Daily, April 4, 2008

54. Li DK, et al, "A population-based prospective cohort study of personal exposure to magnetic fields during pregnancy and the risk of miscarriage," Epidemiology 2002;13:9-20.

55. University of Montreal: Canadian Medical Association Journal: June 2010

56. Endocrinology, June 2003. Human Reproduction, July 2001. American Journal of Obstetrics and Gynecology, January 1999. Theoharis C. Theohardies, MD, PhD, professor of pharmacology, internal medicine and biochemistry, Tufts University School of Medicine, Boston. Calvin J. Hobel, MD, vice chair, department of obstetrics and gynecology, Cedars-Sinai Medical Center, Los Angeles; professor of obstetrics and gynecology, professor of pediatrics, University of California, Los Angeles, School of Medicine.

57. Assay of thyroid hormones and related substances. Last revised by Carol Spenser, Ph D February 6, 2004. www.thyroidmanager.org

58. Roberto Negro, MD et. Al., "Increased Miscarriage Rate in Thyroid Antibody Negative Women with TSH Levels between 2.5 and 5.0 in the First Trimester of Pregnancy," Endocrine Society 92nd Annual Meeting,Absract OR37-4, Endocrine Reviews, Supplement 1, June 2010, 31[3] S2518

59. Am J Obstet Gynecol 2003;188:1241-3

60. Centenary Institute: Journal of Immunology: December 2009

61. Carin A Koelman, Audrey B.C Coumans, et al. Correlation between oral sex and a low incidence of preeclampsia: a role for soluble HLA in seminal fluid?

62. John D Meeker et al. Urinary phthalate metabolites in relation to pre-term birth in Mexico City. Environmental Health Perspectives 16th June 2009

63. Halldorsson TI et al. Intake of artificially sweetened soft drinks and risk of pre-term delivery: a prospective cohort study in 59,334 Danish pregnant women .Am J Clin Nutr. 2010 Sep;92(3):626-33.

64. MJA Volume 184 number 7 April 3 2006

65. It seems the fertility clock ticks for men, too NY Times February 27, 2007

66. Schmatz M et al. Maternal obesity: the interplay between inflammation, mother and fetus Journal of Perinatology 2009;aop:10.1038/jp.2009.182

67. Mills et al. Maternal obesity and congenital heart defects: a population based study.

68. Am J Clin Nutr (April 7, 2010). doi:10.3945/ajcn.2009.28865

69. Nelson SM, Fleming RF. Hum Reprod 2007;22(4):912-91

70. Catalano P. Management of obesity in pregnancy Obstet Gynecol 2007;109(2):419-433

71. Jensen TK, Hjollund NJI. BMJ 1998;317(7157):505-510

72. Muthusami K, et al. Fertil Steril 2005;84(4):919-24

73. Hatch EE, Bracken MB (1993). Association of delayed conception with caffeine consumption. American Journal of Epidemiology, 138(12), 1082-092

74. Pollard I Women & Health 2000;30(3):1-23

75. Florack EI, et al. Prev Med 1994;23(2):175-180

76. Schmid TE, et al. Human Reproduction 2007;22(1):180-187

77. www.urmc.rochester.edu

78. Second hand smoke exposure during pregnancy causes permanent genetic damage in newborns. University of Pittsburgh Schools of the Health Sciences

79. Vine MF, et al. Fertil Steril 1996;65(4):835-42

80. Pollard I Women & Health 2000;30(3):1-23

81. Chavarro, J. et al. Dietary fatty acid intakes and the risk of ovulatory infertility Am J Clin Nutr 2007;85:231-7

82. Austrian Agency for Health and Food Safety, 11 November 2008.

83. Avoid stress and exercise lots during pregnancy 2nd December, 2008 www.news-medical.net

84. Gudmundsdottir SL, et al. Physical activity and fertility in women: the North-Trondelag health study. Hum Reprod 2009;24:3196-3204

85. De Souza MJ, et al. High frequency of LPD and anovulation in recreational women runners: blunted elevation in FSH observed during luteal-follicular transition. J Clin Endocrinol Metab 1998;83:4220-4232

86. Hafez B, et al. Arch Andrology 2004;50(4):207-238

87. G. Can we do more to reduce the burden of cancer? ACNEM 27(2), 2008

88. Steegers EAP. Begin at the beginning: some reflections on future periconceptual and obstetric care and research in the Netherlands. Eur Clinics Obstet Gynecol 2005

89. Preconceptional Folate Supplementation and the Risk of Spontaneous Pre-term Birth: A Cohort Study www.marchofdimes.com

90. Patrick L. Iodine deficiency and therapeutic considerations. Altern Me Rev 2008 Jun;13(2):116-127

91. Li M, et al. Are Australian children iodine deficient? Results of the Australian National Iodine Nutrition Study. Med J Aust 2006 Feb 20;184(4):165-169

92. Shah D, Sachdev HP. Zinc deficiency in pregnancy and fetal outcome. Nutr Rev. 2006;64(1):15-30

93. Henmi H, Endo T, Kitajima Y, et al. Effects of ascorbic acid supplementation on serum progesterone levels in patients with a luteal phase defect. Fertil Steril 2003;80:459–61.

94. Bayer R. Treatment of infertility with vitamin E. Int J Fertil 1960;5:70–8.

95. Vitamin D can aid fertility. 11th November, 2008 www.telegraph.co.uk

96. Vitamin D levels predict IVF reproductive success. 3rd August, 2009 www.orgyn.com

97. Simopoulos AP. Omega-3 Fatty acids in inflammation and autoimmune diseases. J Am Coll Nutr. 2002 Dec;21(6):495-505.

98. Camargo A, Ruano J, Fernandez JM, Parnell LD, Jimenez A, Santos-Gonzalez M, Marin C, Perez-Martinez P, Uceda M, Lopez-Miranda J, Perez-Jimenez F. Gene expression changes in mononuclear cells from patients with metabolic syndrome after acute intake of phenol-rich virgin olive oil. BMC Genomics. 2010 Apr 20;11(1):253

99. Phillips KP, et al. J Toxicol Environ Health B Crit Rev, part B 2008;11:188-220

100. Mlynarcikova A, et al. Endocr Regul 2005;39(1):21-32

101. CDC's Third National Report on Human Exposure to Environmental Chemicals

102. Hugo ER, et al. Environ Health Perspec 2008;116(12):1642-1647

103. Sugiura-Ogasawara M. Ozaki Y et al. Hum Reprod 2005;20(8):2325-2329

104. Challenged Conceptions: Environmental Chemicals and Infertility. Stanford University School of Medicine October 2005

105. Dolinoy DC et al. Maternal nutrient supplementation counteracts bisphenol A induced DNA hypomethylation in early development. PNAS

106. Phillips KP, et al. J Toxicol Environ Health B Crit Rev, Part B 2008;11:188-220

107. Tiemann U Reprod Toxic 2008;25:316-326

108. Wennborg H, et al. Occup Environ Med 2001;58:225-231

109. Triche EW, et al. Semin Perinat 2007;31(4):240-242

110. California Breast Cancer Research Program. Identifying gaps in breast cancer research. Section 1. Physical environment. Chapter B. Pollutants 3. Brominated flame retardants

111. Cherry N, et al. Occup Environ Med 2008 Apr 16

112. Soldin, Offie. Thyroid Function Testing in Pregnancy and Thyroid Disease: Trimester Specific Reference Intervals. Therapeutic Drug Monitor, volume 28, No. 1, February 2006

113. Assay of thyroid hormones and related substances. Carole Spenser, PhD. February 6, 2004 www.thyroidmanager.org

114. New threshold for gestational diabetes Australian Doctor 1st March 2010

115. McLachlan RI, de Kretser DM. Male infertility: The case for continued research. Med J Aust. 2001;174(3):116-7

116. European Society For Human Reproduction And Embryology: June 2005

117. Meniru GI. Cambridge Guide to Infertility Management and Assisted Reproduction. Cambridge University Press, 2001

118. Lefievr L et al. Reproduction 2007;133:675-684

119. Aitken RJ et al. Soc Reprod Fertil Suppl 2007;65:81-92

120. Shamsi MB et al. Indian J Med Res 2008;127:115-123

121. Shamsi MB et al. Indian J Med Res 2008;127:115-123

122. Aitken RJ et al. Soc Reprod Fertil Suppl 2007;65:81-92

123. E.Carlsen, A.Giwereman, N.Keiding and N.E.Skakkebaek, (1992). British Medical Journal 305,609-613

124. R.M.Sharpe, Current Evidence- Another DDT Connection, Nature, vol. 375, 15th June 1995

125. B.Martin and M.Day, New scientist- This week- fresh alarm over threatened sperm, Jan 97 page 5

126. American Society for Reproductive Medicine

127. Krassas GE, et al. Male reproductive function in relation with thyroid alterations. Best Pract Res Clin Endocrinol Metab 2004;18(2):183-95

128. Carani C, et al. Multicentre study on the prevalence of sexual symptoms in male hypo and hyperthyroid patients. J Clin Endocrinol Metab 2005;90(12):6472-9

129. Ruby HN, et al. Body mass index and fertility. Human Reproduction Vol.22, No.9 pp 2488-2493, 2007

130. The Fertility Society of Australia

131. Fertil Steril 2009;92:1318-1325

132. Hauser et al. DNA damage in human sperm is related to urinary levels of phthalate monoester and oxidative metabolites. Hum Reprod 22(3):688-95

133. Sakaue, M, S Ohsako, R Ishimura, S Kurosawa, M Kurohmaru, Y Hayashi, Y Aoki, J Yonemoto and C Tohyama. 2001. Bisphenol-A Affects Spermatogenesis in the Adult Rat Even at a Low Dose. Journal of Occupational Health 43:185 -190.

134. Kutteh, W., Chao, C., Ritter, J., Byrd, W. Vaginal lubricants for the infertile couple: effect on sperm activity. International journal of fertility and menopausal studies 41(4), 1996.

135. H J Chi et al. Reproduction 2008;23(5):1023-1028

136. Akinloye O et al. Biological Trace Element Research 2005;104:9-18

137. Scott R et al. Br J Urol 1998;82:76-80

138. Tikkiwal M et al. Ind J Phys Pharm 1987;31:30-34

139. Carpino et al. Molecular Human Reproduction 1999;5(4):338-341

140. Kessopoulou E et al. Fert & Steril 1995;64(4):825-31

141. Oshio et al. Journal of Nutritional Science and Vitaminology 1992;53(2):95-101

142. Boxmeer JC et al. J Androl 2007;28(4):521-7

143. Wong et al. The New England Journal of Medicine 2002;344(15):1172-1173

144. Suleimen SA et al. Jour Androl 1996;17:530-37

145. Greco E et al. Journal of Andrology 2005;26(3):349-353

146. Khademi A et al. Iranian Journal of Reproductive Medicine 2004;2(2):65-69

147. Prien et al. Molecular Human Reproduction 1999;5(4):331-337

148. How to make sperm better. Australian Doctor. 1st July, 2009

149. How to make sperm better. Australian Doctor. 1st July, 2009

References

150. Dr Alastair Sutcliffe, Prof. Michael Ludwig, Outcome of assisted reproduction. The Lancet Volume 370, issue 9584, July 2007

151. Birth, 3rd September 2010.

152. European Society of Human Genetics

153. Carter M. Owen; James H. Segars. Imprinting disorders and assisted reproductive technology 12/21/2009; Semin Reprod Med. 2009;27(5):417-428. © 2009

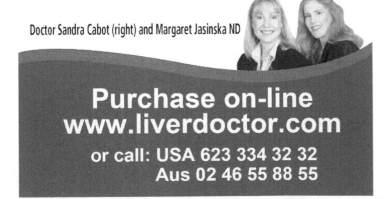

This is what you will find at:

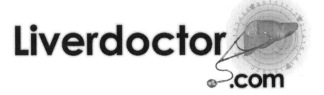

Liverdoctor.com

Holistic medical information

Well researched and up-to-date information to help you in your daily life
Informative on-line information to assist you look after your health and weight

Free liver check up test

Take this liver check up and receive private & confidential feedback on
the state of your liver and general health - www.liverdoctor.com/liver-check

Health supplements

Including Doctor Cabot's Livatone Plus capsules to support optimal liver function

On-line shopping

Sandra Cabot MD has a excellent range of health products and publications

On-line help from Dr Cabot's Team

Confidential and expert help from Dr Cabot's highly trained nutritionists and
naturopaths. Simply email us at ehelp@liverdoctor.com

Free LIVERISH newsletter

Register on-line for the free LIVERISH nesletter at www.liverdoctor.com/newsletter

Love you liver and live longer

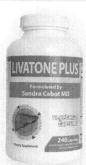

I am so glad I have been able to assist thousands of people to regain their health and vitality.

Sandra Cabot

Dr Sandra Cabot MBBS DRCOG

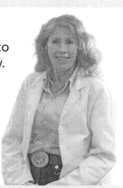

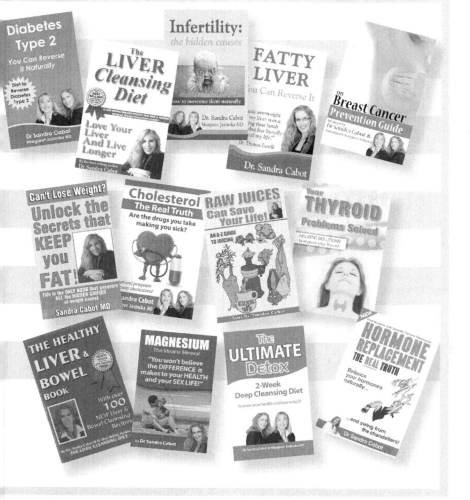